SLÁINTE!

THE GOOD HEALTH GUIDE
Alternative and Complementary Medicine

SLÁINTE!

THE GOOD HEALTH GUIDE
Alternative and Complementary Medicine

Edited by Susanna Hassett

WOLFHOUND PRESS

© 1990 Susanna Hassett and individual contributors
First published 1990
WOLFHOUND PRESS
68 Mountjoy Square,
Dublin 1.

British Library Cataloguing in Publication Data
Hassett, Susanna
      Sláinte: the good health guide
      1. Alternative Medicine
      I. Title
      615.5

ISBN 0-86327-252-5

Cover design: Jan de Fouw
Illustrations: Cathy Dineen
Typesetting: Phototype-Set Ltd.
Printed by: The Guernsey Press Ltd.

Contents

for Pauline Daly and Sandra Calvet
and

> 'For all of you who must discover,
> For all of you who understand,
> For having found the path of others,
> You find a very special hand.
> And it is a holy thing, and it is a precious time,
> And it is the only way.'

(from *Bright Blue Rose* by Jimmy McCarthy.)

ACKNOWLEDGEMENTS AND THANKS

To all who contributed articles, advice, loans of books and articles, long technical discussions, lists of association members, names of practitioners, insights and support — my heartfelt thanks. It's been great.

To Dr. Brian Kennedy for detailed reading and comments, special thanks.

To Mary Grant, of Lifespring in Belfast, I am especially grateful for providing the opportunity of including practitioners north and south of the border. Mary Grant and Lifespring produced the *Natural Guide to Health and Healing*, for N. Ireland, in 1988.

Thanks to Louis-Guy, Marie-Christine, Maura, Paddy, Fintan, John, Josie, Mary Kelly and Fin Costello, Maria, Theo, Sarah and Derek, for friendship, guidance, and therapy.

To Clodagh Corcoran and Mary Gallagher for the sponges in the corner.

To Ron and Miriam, without whose chauffeuring of children to and from school I would not have had the time to do it.

To Bernadette, for baby-sitting and keeping order in the household.

To Wolfhound Press for anchorage, again, my thanks.

To my first family.

Above all to Tom Daly, Fionn and Brian, my love and thanks for your love and patience.

Editor's Introduction

This book has been written with two objectives in mind: Firstly, to help people who need healthcare to find the method and practitioner that suits them. Secondly, for practitioners of Medicine, mainstream and otherwise. I would hope that it contributes to the understanding of what is available in Ireland and what needs to become available.

The structure of *Sláinte*: Each category of Healing is followed by a relevant list of practitioners. Some of the articles have been written by practitioners, others by myself with the help of professionals. We have aimed both to outline the principles of each method and to give the 'feel' of each area covered.

I have found, during my own illnesses, that different approaches work at different times. At one time I needed to talk about my feelings, at another to rest and be healed spiritually, at yet another to work with a technique such as reflexology, acupuncture or osteopathy, and so on. I hope that *Sláinte* will help people who are ill or who care for the ill to choose more surely. Some of my experiences are discussed in the main text of the book.

The Status of Practitioners Listed

Practitioners listed in this book belong, for the most part to a professional body and most of the listings have been supplied by such bodies. Where professional bodies do not as yet exist, and where practitioners have chosen individually not to join, our policy has been to list all practitioners, stating their individual qualifications. Readers are therefore advised that, since no list of legally qualified practitioners exists in Ireland, they should choose a practitioner or practitioners whose qualifications satisfy them. No responsibility will be accepted by the author or the publishers for any form or instance of malpractice by practitioners listed here.

Also because there are no associations for some of the methods covered here, it is inevitable that not all practitioners are listed. The fact that a practitioner is not listed is in no way intended as a reflection or judgement on his or her work. Any practitioner who is not listed and who would like to be included in future editions is invited to send details to the publisher.

Selecting a Practitioner

We offer the following suggestions: The diversity of certificates and titles that exist make these a variable guide to quality, but do give an indication of practitioners' levels of training. In addition to satisfying yourself as to a practitioner's qualifications and experience, you should choose a practitioner who carries Professional Indemnity and Public Liability Insurance. Where possible, this information is given in *Sláinte*, but insurance of this type has only recently been made available to practitioners. As a result there may now be more practitioners insured than at the time of publication.

Word of mouth is a good guide to practitioners; successful treatment is its own advertisement.

In general, one of the strong and appealing features of parallel medicine is that its practitioners work with the whole person, that they will listen to and take account of the client's needs and situation. If you feel that a practitioner is too brusque, or is rushing people through without giving sufficient attention, complain or go elsewhere. As will be seen on reading the articles in this book, both diagnosis and treatment in most forms of parallel medicine demand the client's involvement.

If you feel that the treatment is costing too much, point this out. It is normal that more than one session will be needed, but treatment should have a beginning, a middle and an end in sight. If treatment is required over a long period, this should in most cases be clear at the outset and the terms of payment should be agreed. Since parallel medicine is not recognised by the State, its practitioners do not receive a fee for treating Medical Card Holders. However, many offer a concession to the unemployed or low-waged, and some carry a proportion of non-paying patients. Look around for a practitioner you can afford, or one who may be willing to barter! Do NOT abuse this facility where you find it!

Training courses for those who wish to learn about preventative care, natural medicines and techniques that can be used in the home are becoming more widely available. It is well worth attending such a course and thus avoiding the necessity to call for medical help for minor ailments.

If you have a young family, as I do, and even if you don't, look for a practitioner who will do house-calls in times of crisis. I am concerned, as many other parents are, at the health risks involved in repeated antibiotic prescribing by GPs. But equally, an alternative practitioner with a six week waiting list is not much use if you or your children suddenly come down with an illness that demands immediate attention!

Keep your options open. A time may come when you feel you simply have to go to the hospital or take prescribed medication. There is an increase in instances where traditional and parallel medicine are used together, but this may not always be practicable. Practitioners of one may not be willing to co-operate with the other, either on principle or for medical reasons. (My experience has been that GPs are less willing to cooperate with parallel practitioners than vice versa). If possible, identify the merits of each without allowing yourself to be brow-beaten.

Finally, be aware of your state of health without becoming neurotic. Aim to prevent ill-health. Choose your diet with care and exercise regularly. Learn to recognise stress as it arises and to deal with it. If stress seems unavoidable, practice a form of relaxation such as meditation, visualisation, breathing exercises, etc.

1992 and the Regulation of Practitioners

An EC Directive (89/48/EC) has been issued which lays down the system for the recognition of higher education diplomas. It is intended to control the movement of professionals between EC states and is to be implemented by the end of 1992. It is impossible to predict how this will affect the regulation of practitioners inside Ireland. Practitioners within Ireland are encouraged towards self-regulation (see the statement made by Department of Health in Dublin, at the end of this section.)

As well as professional associations for particular therapies there is a body which aims to unite and represent the interests of Irish practitioners of different methods: The Institute of

Alternative Medicine, 6, Martello Tce., Monkstown, Co. Dublin.

Natural Medicines

An allied debate is that about natural medicines which are currently available from wholefood stores and some chemists. The EC Review of Medicines is to be completed by May 1990. Most medicines have already been reviewed. Vitamin and mineral supplements, Herbal, Homoeopathic, and Anthroposophic medicines are presently being reviewed in this country.

Under the Review Scheme, manufacturers can be required to change manufacturing procedures and medicines can be withdrawn pending clinical trials. The cost of implementing these standards and of carrying out clinical trials may be prohibitive to the continued manufacture of some Natural medicines.

Licences will now be required to import the above items for resale, and special regulations and a registration procedure will apply to homoeopathic remedies. Injectible anthroposophic medicines, which fall into this category, cannot be imported for re-sale until these procedures are implemented and three such have recently been temporarily withdrawn. However, doctors can import them on a named-patient basis by applying to the National Drugs Advisory Board. Homoeopathic physicians can import homoeopathic remedies without a licence, for the purpose of dispensing them to patients. Essential oils, used in aromatherapy will also come under review.

The Natural Medicines Society was formed in Ireland in 1989 to help ensure that procedures implemented are not overly restrictive to the availability of natural medicines. The society is open to all to join and can be contacted by writing to: The Natural Medicines Society, P.O. Box 2428, Dublin 6.

Conclusion

Natural Medicines and parallel medicine are not available in this country under the General Medical Scheme and so their use is restricted to those who can afford them. Whilst in growing demand they are far from being freely available.

There is still a huge gap between dissatisfaction with mainstream medicine and finding a satisfactory alternative. I hope that this book goes some way towards closing that gap, and that people will join together to close it even further.

Mainstream medicine is clearly not meeting the needs we have. The medical industry often promotes and dismisses different treatments in response to economic strategy. The New Age search is an attempt to find relief from the mainly psychological stresses of modern society. People are looking for personal experiences, personal contact and personal development. The concept of wholeness is central to alternative medical practise. It is a word that resonates in writings about healing, from the *Yellow Emperor's Compendium of Internal Medicine* to the *Bible*. It is the demand of every sick person — make me 'whole'. And it is a word that disappeared from serious Science some time ago and was replaced by analysis. Analysis has its place, but synthesis or catharsis must follow . . .

The concept that unites the methods of medical practice included here is that of The Vital Force. In medical terms, The Vital Force is that aspect of the living creature which keeps the body healthy and which works to maintain and restore health. It can be felt in others and experienced in oneself, and this book is about those medical practices which recognise and work with it. Finally, although many are concerned to legitimise alternative medicine by using scientific and medical terms, it must be said that the concept of Universal Love underlies the concept of The Vital Force and in my opinion, healing is incomplete without that Love.

Sláinte romhat,
Susanna Hassett.

A request to readers
In the interest of promoting national regulation and recognition of practitioners of alternative medicine, the editor and publisher of this book recommend that readers should send a letter to the Secretary, Department of Health, Hawkins House, Dublin 2, requesting that action be taken. Reputable practitioners in the field have requested Department of Health initiative in this matter but have been informed that the Department's function is rather to respond to public demand. Letters from readers to the Department and local politicians may be the only way to encourage movement towards regulatory control. Finally, we welcome entries for future editions of this Directory. Please write to The Editor, Sláinte, Wolfhound Press, 68 Mountjoy Square, Dublin 1.

Alternative Medicine
A Statement from the Department of Health, Dublin

Practitioners of alternative medicine are not subject to any formal process of regulation or recognition by the Department of Health and are free to engage in the practice of medicine provided the persons concerned do not represent themselves as registered medical practitioners. Those engaged in practice are, of course, subject to common law provisions relating to matters of safety. Officials of the Department have met with representative bodies of practitioners of alternative medicine on a number of occasions. The representative bodies have been concerned for some time about the issues of control of standards and codes of practice in the area of alternative medicine. The Department has encouraged the representative bodies to consider a system of self regulation in relation to matters of training, recognition and advertising.

At present, the Department is drafting legislation for the registration of certain designated health professionals (e.g. radiographers, speech therapists, etc.).

The Department's view is that relative to the position of the designated health professions for inclusion under the imminent system of registration, those engaged in the practice of alternative medicine are at an early stage of developing structured training programmes, and introducing standards and codes of practice. However, the proposed legislation is being prepared on such a basis that the framework of registration could be extended to other groups where it is considered appropriate to do so.

Chapter One

HERBALISM

I would like to thank Sean Boylan and Sylvia Voss for their part in this article.

Herbal Medicines have been in use through the ages, declining in popularity with the growth of cities and urban living. Their use in Europe was virtually eliminated by the rapid growth of the pharmaceutical industry and the flood of synthetic drugs produced. Many such drugs emulate the properties and action of herbal remedies on the human body — for instance, anyone with an awareness of heroin addiction will know of synthetic opiates as well as those produced from the opium poppy.

As medical science turned its attention to the task of identifying specific diseases with a specific definable feature or features, research projects that sought to identify the active ingredient of existing herbal remedies mushroomed. Of course, the extent to which any substance can be seen as 'active' on the human body depends on the instrumentation used. Substances present in herbal remedies in quantities too small to measure were deemed irrelevant to the curative process. Substances identified as 'active' were produced in vast quantities, from plant extracts, and usually by artificial means. Medicines and healthcare were industrialised and socialised and although the benefits of that are undeniable so are the negative side-effects such as the use of artificial preservatives on the grand scale, hazardous work practices and industrial pollution.

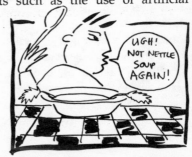

The Whole Plant

In herbal medicine it is traditional that the whole

plant is curative. The leaves, flowers, stem and root may act in different ways, but all are important and must be used whole, together or separately. It is also traditional that wherever possible, plants grown in the same region as the sick person should be used for treatment. While there may be more of one substance than any other in a plant, it is the combination of all substances that is curative. Similarly, a person may not respond well to plants grown in foreign climates which would be likely to contain substances or a mixture of substances varying in quality from those in the home environment to which the body is accustomed.

Studies of the side-effects of synthetic drugs and artificial foodstuffs serve, ironically, to illustrate this point. It has been found that many allergic-type conditions result from the body's inability to digest artificial substances which have a slightly different molecular structure to the natural product. The human digestive system and the enzymes in particular, match exactly the molecular structures in natural foodstuffs, and are irritated and often sickened by the synthetic variety. In effect, the body is dealing with a different and unfamiliar substance! Where a food or medicinal substance is whole, its ingredients can be readily absorbed by the human body. (This point is expanded in the chapter Diet and Nutrition). For now, it serves to illustrate the wisdom of herbalists in emphasising the importance of all of the properties of plants.

Laboratory Testing

Following the world-wide distribution of drugs such as thalidomide, DES and others, which deformed, damaged or killed thousands of people, scientific testing of drugs has been much discussed. Laboratory tests of new drugs, mainly carried out on animals, is now mandatory before a new drug can be released on the open market. Experimentation with drugs on animals has been widely discredited not only for the cruelty to the animals used, but also because the effects of a drug on one species does not exactly carry over to another species. Now, drugs which have passed a certain stage of laboratory testing are often tried out on human volunteers — often poverty-stricken or desperate volunteers.

Those threatened by the growth in the use of herbal and other natural remedies now seek to impose regulations on their production and distribution. Internationally, it is sought to impose testing on herbal remedies in laboratories owned or to be established by the pharmaceutical industry. In Ireland it is sought to restrict their importation and sale to those agents and outlets already dealing with drugs.

The rules of evidence in scientific testing do not, unfortunately, seem capable of acknowledging the fact that something that has been used to successfully treat illness over generations has already been tested and proven. Or if it is acknowledged, it is sought to own a remedy or remedies and to restrict to experts what was once folklore.

The witches of the woods were the generation of herbalists prior to this, and we all know what happened to them! Practising herbalists and particularly those who have learned the craft from an older practitioner in the traditional way, are, it seems, also under attack, this time in the form of written examinations of their skill and laboratory testing of their cures.

The Test of Time

Herbal remedies have been discovered over the ages of history and tested over that timespan. Everyone remembers back to their childhood when they used to squeeze a dock leaf over a nettle sting and they in turn show this magic to their own children. But sadly, we have forgotten the properties of the herbs we use in cooking, scorn nettle soup, and admire the lawn that has no weeds, only grass. Although Schools of Herbalism or Phytotherapy (plant therapy) now exist, it is regrettable that the understanding of the simple properties of common herbs is no longer widespread.

In my opinion, it is this understanding and not the 'professionalisation' or 'industrialisation' of herbal medicine that will ensure safe practices in its production, use and sale. There is no doubt that herbal preparations can be injurious to health if improperly administered, and the field of herbalism requires great knowledge and skill. However, there is much in herbalism that is easily accessible — plants that can be grown in the garden or found growing wild and that can be used in mild illnesses. Many such plants are also extraordinarily high in mineral and vitamin content and their inclusion in one's diet can be preventative of illness. Substance abuse is a problem of our time, but one that would surely be alleviated rather than worsened by popular understanding of the properties of herbs and thence of nature.

An Irish Herbalist

Notwithstanding the competition from synthetic drugs, and partly because of dissatisfaction with them, herbalists in this country are still much sought after and recognised for their cures. Sean Boylan is one herbalist, based in Co. Meath. At his clinic, there are always people waiting — some who have appointments and some who don't. A lot of people just turn up, from as far away as Co. Mayo and are amazed at the number of others who have done the same. Those who have appointments are naturally a bit put out by this, but after the initial surprise, people tend to wait, for hours sometimes, to be seen. Sean himself admits that it is difficult to meet the demand and to follow up cases in detail, and for this reason works with two others who have been trained by him and elsewhere and who have now joined him in his practice.

In the fashion of the traditional herbalist, intuition goes hand in hand with technical knowledge of the human anatomy in diagnosing and prescribing for a client. The questions asked of a patient are reminiscent of the detail demanded in a Homoeopathic consultation, while the examination is similar to that of an Osteopath. Sean Boylan emphasises above all an understanding of people and the ability to see and stimulate natural vitality — by working on the client's attitude and feelings as well as by prescribing a remedy.

While much can be learned and taught in a College of Phytotherapy, and while cures can be classified and analysed 'scientifically', an understanding of the properties of herbs involves as well a sense of their essential properties and an ability to match these with the essential qualities of the patient. This can only be acquired by contact with herbs while they are growing and being harvested and by an openness towards all nature, including human nature.

It is Sean Boylan's suggestion that anyone interested in herbalism should begin with a few, by growing them at home and gradually using them in more and more ways — in cooking, for teas, in poultices and powders, and in the bath.

Parsley, Sage, Rosemary and Thyme

Parsley is under the dominion of Mercury. The distilled water of parsley is traditionally given to babies who are fretting with wind in the stomach and also to elderly people with the same complaint. Its leaves, when laid on inflamed or swollen eyes, provide ease. Fried in butter, it will ease a woman's breasts when swollen and hard with milk, and will also remove bruises.

Sage is claimed by Jupiter, and is good for the liver and the blood. It is most commonly used as a tea to prevent and ease coughs and colds during the Winter months. It can easily be hung and dried in a warm, airy part of the house and later kept in an airtight container. It tastes as good as regular tea and a little honey can be added for the sweet tooth.

Rosemary is ruled by the Sun, and it is in the house of the celestial Ram. Burning Rosemary in a room, or in the whole house, clears and corrects the air. The leaves can be used in the bath as a general tonic and Rosemary makes an excellent hair-conditioner.

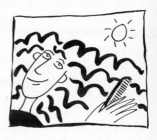

Thyme is a herb of Venus. It purges the body of phlegm and is an excellent remedy for shortness of breath. It mildly and safely assists women in labour and helps to bring away the after-birth. It is excellent for anyone troubled with gout.

Listing of Herbalists

Cork:
Alan Chaytor-Grubb, Cork Clinic of Herbal Medicine, 5, Tuckey St., Cork. Tel. 021-275638
Meath:
Sean Boylan, Edenmore,Dunboyne, Co. Meath. Tel.01-255250
Mary Hutton, address as above, also Reflexology.
Martin O'Reagan, address as above, also Therapeutic Massage.
Tipperary:
Christine Maxwell,Dulcamara, Modeshill, Mullinahone, Co. Tipperary. Tel. 052-53256. B.Sc., Dip. in Phytotherapy, also Homoeopathic and Anthroposophical Medicine.
Tyrone:
Robert Elliott, Chartered Herbalist, B.Sc., 23, Westland Rd., Cookstown, Co. Tyrone BT80 8BX. Tel. Cookstown 66454/62138

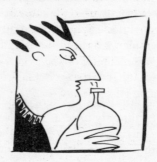

Aromatherapy

I would like to thank Mary Cavanagh and Mary Anderson for their help with this article.

Aromatherapy is a treatment designed to help, cure or heal by the correct use or application of pure essential oils obtained from plants. These oils are extracted from the leaves, stems and flowers of plants from many parts of the world and are used for the treatment of physical, emotional and spiritual ills by Aromatherapists.

The healing properties of plants are concentrated in essential oils which can be used in the following ways:
— by inhalation from a tissue or cloth handkerchief
— by adding 6 to 8 drops to a bath
— by adding a few drops to a small bowl of water placed over a radiator

— by using an oil-burner. These are available from most whole-food shops. A few drops of oil are added to a small amount of water and this is placed over a small candle or night-light, releasing the aroma of the oil.
— massage of the body, using a few drops of an essential oil mixed in a fine carrier oil.

Professional Aromatherapy treatment entails a thorough consultation helped by using the Reflex techniques on the feet (see Chapter 7, Reflexology), to enable the correct essential oils to be chosen and blended to cater for the needs of the individual requiring help. These oils are then mixed in a fine carrier oil and applied to the body and face. Specialised massage movements are used to stimulate the circulation, improve movement of the lymph and therefore the removal of its associated toxins from the body. The muscles become relaxed enabling the essential oils to penetrate the skin and be carried round with the increased circulation to all parts of the body. The treatment is finished with a very relaxing facial and scalp massage.

An Aromatherapy consultation and massage will last for an hour or more and is one of *the* most relaxing experiences ever. Tension just melts away as the therapist massages the whole body and the aroma of the oils adds to the feeling of relaxation of mind and body. The massage technique used by Aromatherapists combines stimulation of some of the pressure points from Shiatsu with a technique known as *effleurage*, which is a gentle circular motion, and, of course, essential oils in a carrier, or base oil are used.

Aromatherapy is used as a treatment for a wide range of illnesses and is particularly effective for conditions that are stress-related. As well as treating conditions that have already developed, Aromatherapy can be used as a preventative technique — an Aromatherapy massage every month will help to avoid the build up of tension and add to one's sense of well-being. Aromatherapy is suitable for every age-group, but it is advisable to consult a qualified practitioner before treating serious illnesses at home and before treating children, who require smaller amounts of milder oils than adults. Some people are put off by the idea of having to undress, or by the idea of a whole body massage, but any reservations of this type are guaranteed to disappear after one treatment! I would particularly recommend Aromatherapy massage for the aches and pains of the elderly — older friends and family members of mine have found tremendous benefit from regular treatment.

Essential oils

Essential oils are becoming increasingly popular as part of the First Aid kit at home, some helpful oils are listed below:

Lavender is perhaps the most popular and versatile oil of all. It blends well with other essential oils, aids relaxation and heals many skin conditions. Four drops of Lavender added to a dessertspoon of a carrier oil, such as almond or grapeseed oil, can relax away a tension headache when massaged gently into the back of the neck and the temples. Used neat on a burn, it will stop pain and prevent blistering and swelling. Similarly, it can be used on cuts to assist the healing process and prevent infection. In an oil burner or in a bowl of water placed over a radiator it freshens the air, creating a relaxing atmosphere.

Rosemary is invigorating, refreshing, it sharpens the memory and enlivens the mind. It is used to stimulate the circulation and mixed with Juniper oil to treat cellulite and fluid retention. It is renowned as a hair conditioner and as a cure for scalp conditions. A little whiff from a tissue is great in the office or when studying.

Geranium is good to add to the bath after a hard day, relaxing the body and refreshing the mind. Run the bath and when full, add 6 to 8 drops. Swirl the water to mix the oil. Get in and relax for ten to fifteen minutes.

Basil is used to treat sinus problems. 3 to 5 drops on a tissue will give relief when inhaled. Sinus problems can also be treated with Basil oil in a traditional steam bath; add a few drops to a bowl of boiling water, cover the head and basin with a large towel and inhale. Repeat twice daily for a few days.

List of Practitioners

The Natural Therapy Centre (NTC), Dun Laoghaire is the accredited Training School in Ireland for the Shirley Price Aromatherapy Diploma Course. The Shirley Price Diploma Course includes training in Reflex Zone Techniques, study of the properties and uses of the essential oils and a grounding in physiology and anatomy. The NTC also offers a six-week introductory course in basic massage and the healing properties of essential oils. Courses in Cork and Dundalk are arranged.

Further information is available from: Mary Cavanagh, The Natural Therapy Centre, 12, Tivoli Tce. South, Dun Laoghaire, Co. Dublin. Tel. 01-809505. Holders of the NTC Diploma are listed below.

Clare:
Annette Gardiner, Ennis, Co. Clare. Tel. 065-21557.
Dublin:
Lucy Carroll, Harold's Cross, Dublin 6. Tel.(messages) 01-809595;
Mary Cavanagh, The Natural Therapy and Yoga Centre, 12, Tivoli Tce., Dun Laoghaire, Co. Dublin. Tel. 01-809505;
Bernadette Jewell, Clondalkin, Dublin 22. Tel. 01-573819;
Sara Power, Terenure, Dublin 12. Tel. 01-909915;
Maura Purcell, Templeogue, Dublin 6. Tel. 01-903137;
Barbara Rocks, Walkinstown, Dublin 12. Tel. 01-551456;
Celia Slevin, Terenure, Dublin 6. Tel. 01-900195.
Kerry:
Claire Chamberlain, nr Kenmare, Killarney, Co. Kerry. Tel. 064-84290;
Mary O' Donoghue, Tralee, Co. Kerry. Tel. 066-22857.
Mayo:
Martina Barrett, Castlebar, Co. Mayo. Tel. Castlebar 23161.
Wexford:
Shirley Copeland, "Kellar", Maudlinstown, Wexford;
Kate Murphy, Enniscorthy, Co. Wexford. Tel. 054-33484;

Courses:
Mary Anderson, Hamilton House, Trafalgar Tce., Monkstown, Co. Dublin. Tel. 01-803635. Mary Anderson practises and teaches Aromatherapy. Details of Aromatherapists who have trained at her school are available from the following numbers :

Mary Collins, Tel. 021-274130;
Geri Halpin, Tel. 041-35565;
Mary Anderson, as above.
Maureen Hammond, Tel. 01-982402;
Ann Williams Tel. 01-322172.

Independent Practitioners

Dublin:
Mary Berkerey, 88, Richmond Park, Monkstown, Co. Dublin. Tel. 01-843153; Aromatherapy body massage and facials, Reflexology, Natural Skin Care Advice; Susan Gavin, Ballybrack, Co. Dublin. Tel. 01-825151; Melissa Mae, South Circular Road, Dublin 8. Tel. 01-536140; also Auric and Colour Healing, Bach flower Remedies, Nutritional Counselling and Spiritual Psychotherapy.; Justin McKenna, 70, Drimnagh Rd., Dublin 12. Tel. 01-559973; Maureen O'Malley, 4, Cabinteely Park, Dublin. Tel. 01-857078

Cork:
Julie Reed, Sycamore, Droum, Leap, Co. Cork.

Wicklow:
Avril Bailey, 169, Redford Pk., Greystones, Co. Wicklow. Tel. 01-877369; also Reflexology.

Northern Ireland Practitioners

Vera Boyd, Bangor, Co. Down. Tel.0247-270626; Mary Grant, Lifespring, 111, Cliftonville Rd., Belfast BT14. Tel. 0232-753658; Anne Munro, Lifetree, 37, Spencer Rd., Derry BT47 1DQ. Tel. Derry 42865; also Kinesiology, Bach Flower Remedies, Medical Herbalist, Allergy Testing, Remedial Massage, Healthfood shop; Mary Grant Associates offers a comprehensive training programme in Kairos Aromatherapy — Basic and Post Graduate, including Reflexology, Massage, (Swedish, Neuro Muscular, Lymphatic drainage, Shiatsu), Anatomy and Physiology.

The Bach Flower Remedies

by John McLoughlin

John McLoughlin *is a Natural Healer practising Acupuncture, Remedial massage, giving Dietary Counselling and using Herbal remedies and the Bach Flower Remedies.*

When Dr. Edward Bach, a talented doctor, bacteriologist and pathologist, gave up his very successful Harley Street practice, his contemporaries were shocked. On learning that this man, who they regarded as a genius, had not only walked away from a prestigious and moneyed position, but had done so to go pick flowers in the wilds of Wales, they were certain the genius had turned madman. Bach had turned alright but it was not an overnight turn. Some thirteen years previously, he had collapsed and suffered a severe haemorrhage and was told that he had a rare disease and

three months to live. He had long been dissatisfied with the orthodox medicine he was practising, especially disliking the side effects of the drugs being used. Herbal medicine with its use of safer, more natural and gentle remedies was attracting him. The news of his death-sentence acted as a catalyst that spurred him on to follow his intuition and in 1930 he closed the door on his medical practice and went in search of his herbal healers.

Bach made a miraculous recovery not only outliving his prognosed three months but also enjoying better health that at any other time in his life. He became absolutely convinced that for the body to be healthy, a happy state of being was vital, and that if an unhappy state of mind was allowed to persist it would sooner or later result in a distortion of the vital energy and produce a physical illness. By changing the underlying mental disharmony, equilibrium would be restored and the body would regain its health. As alternative approaches to medicine have become more popular in recent times, this concept of the nature of illness has also become more widely accepted. Back in 1930, when things were a little more conservative much of Bach's work was ridiculed by his contemporaries. Undiscouraged, he continued his work and discovered the wild flowers he used as his remedies. In his book he called them *The Twelve Healers*. In 1934 Bach wrote the following concerning the way his flower remedies work:

'The action of these remedies is to raise our vibrations and open up our channels for the reception of the Spiritual Self; to flood our natures with the particular virtue we need and wash out from us the fault that is causing the harm. They are able like beautiful music or any glorious uplifting thing which gives us inspiration to raise our very natures and bring us nearer to our souls and by that very act to bring us peace and relieve our sufferings. They cure, not by attacking the disease but by flooding our bodies with the beautiful vibrations of our Higher Nature in the presence of which, disease melts away as snow in the sunshine. There is no true healing unless there is a change in outlook, peace of mind and inner-happiness.'

At first this may sound rather improbable, but it actually makes good sense if the basis of Bach's line of thought, which is very similar to Hippocrates and Paracelsus, is understood and accepted. Each believed that every human being has an immortal Soul or Essence that is part of the source of all creation. This Soul has a specific mission, task, destiny or karma to fulfil on this planet and the individual's true life's work is to bring this to full expression. The person also has a mortal personality and a Higher Self which is closely bound up with the soul and may be said to function as a mediator between the soul and the personality. The soul constantly wishes to bring to realisation the higher ideals and qualities such as gentleness, firmness, courage, constancy, wisdom, joyfulness, purposefulness, etc. Now the problem arises when, for whatever reason, the personality goes into conflict with the soul and manifests the opposite or negative aspect of these noble qualities. Defects of mind like pride, cruelty, hatred, self-love, ignorance, greed etc. become the dominant vibrations and produce corresponding defects in the physical body. Bach did not use the physical symptoms to make his diagnosis but based his choice of remedy entirely on the negative mental state. For example if the person was

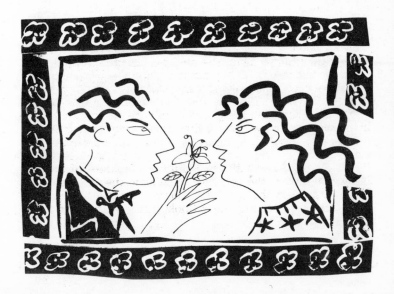

suffering from chronic asthma and on being questioned regarding their mental state said that they generally felt inadequate in the face of responsibility and were easily discouraged then the remedies to be prescribed would be *Elm* and *Gentian*. The state of mind is treated, never the physical symptoms.

Bach used *Mimulus* for any disease whose underlying root was fear; *Clematis* he gave to sleepy, indifferent types whose concentration was poor; *Impatiens* was the remedy for impatient individuals; *Agrimony* for restless tormented minds hidden behind a cheerful facade; *Vervain* for highly strung, highly enthusiastic individuals; *Centaury* for the weak-willed and subservient; *Cerato* for those who constantly seek advice and confirmation from others; *Gentian* for those with a negative outlook. If the keyword is terror, *Rock Rose* is the remedy. *Scleranthus* is for uncertainty and indecision; *Water Violet* for the overly proud and aloof.

Bach Flower Remedies can be used by anyone, anywhere, anytime, without the slightest hesitation or fear. as they are completely harmless and free of side effects. They can be taken in conjunction with other forms of medication or therapies. They are an easily used form of self-healing and the appropriate remedy or combination of remedies can be ascertained by reading the list of mental states associated with each Flower and choosing the one that is most suitable for you. Sometimes it is difficult to be objective about one's mental state and it may be helpful to get the assistance of someone, professional or otherwise, who is familiar with the remedies and their application. Bach Flower Remedies can be found in most whole-food shops and some chemists. Self-help sheets are freely available as well as charts and books on the origin and use of the remedies.

John McLoughlin's Clinic is at 55, Ranelagh, Dublin 6. Tel. 01-757132/971188. (By appointment only).

Chapter Two

ORIENTAL MEDICINE

Traditional Chinese Medicine

by Tom Shanahan, M.A. (Oxon.), C.Ac. (Nanjing)

Tom Shanahan *is a practitioner and teacher of Traditional Chinese Medicine including Acupuncture, and the founder of the Irish College of Traditional Chinese Medicine and the Practitioners Register of Traditional Chinese Medicine.*

Since I will deal elsewhere with the most popularly known branch of Traditional Chinese Medicine (TCM) in the West, namely Acupuncture, I can here turn my attention to the other branches which are much less known, understood or practised in Ireland. In explaining the various aspects of TCM which Chairman Mao accurately describes as a 'treasure house' of knowledge, I would also like to provide a few pointers to the general public on how to recognise a practitioner of TCM. This I shall do within the text itself, as the opportunities present.

Origins and spread of TCM

The origins of TCM stretch back into the mists of time, before history in the form of written records. It is one of the oldest and yet most sophisticated bodies of medicine known to man. In spite of its age-old origins TCM has only become widely known and accepted in the West over the past few decades. In that relatively short time, however, it has gone from strength to strength in terms of patient usage and students wanting to take it up as a professional career.

Safety of TCM

The very fact that TCM is so ancient prompts two further considerations, the first of which is that it must have proved

The Professional Register of Traditional Chinese Medicine

The Register publishes a directory of fully-trained and insured practitioners of Acupuncture and Chinese Medicine who are bound by a code of ethics and a code of practice and are covered by full professional indemnity and public liability insurance (Lloyds).

Details:

The Secretary, 100 Marlborough Road, Dublin 4.
Telephone/Fax: Dublin 216524

Member of the Irish Acupuncture Council
Member of the Institute of Alternative Medicine
Professional Association of the Irish College of Traditional Chinese Medicine

---

The Irish College of Traditional Chinese Medicine

ACUPUNCTURE

Professional Training in Chinese Medicine
Part-Time 3-year Course
Full professional Qualifications
International Insurance (Lloyds)

Details:

The Director, Thomas J. Shanahan,
M.A. (Oxon), Clin. Ac. Cert (Nanjing) China

The Irish College of Traditional Chinese Medicine
100 Marlborough Road, Dublin 4.
Telephone/Fax: Dublin 216524

Teaching Body of the Professional Register of Traditional Chinese Medicine itself to be a thoroughly safe body of medical knowledge and practice not only over the past centuries but over thousands of years. If it had not shown itself to be safe, in terms of literally millions of 'field trials', it would surely have been abandoned long ago. In China today there are well over one thousand million people who are virtually exclusively treated by TCM.

Effectiveness of TCM

The second consideration is similar to the first in that its antiquity suggests not only its safety but also its effectiveness. If TCM did not work it would have been discarded long ago. It is a fact that the self-same herbal prescriptions, to take a representative example here, are used in modern-day TCM surgeries throughout the world as were used over two thousand years ago in China. The antiquity of TCM argues both its safety and effectiveness, presuming that it always is practised exclusively by fully trained experts.

Variety in TCM

The third distinguishing feature of TCM is its wide range of therapeutic options. It has several ways of treating illness and improving or increasing health. Unlike its Western counterpart, sometimes referred to as 'technological' or 'modern' medicine, TCM has at its command totally distinct types of treatment that can be ideally suited to every individual patient's needs. It does not propose a 'pill for every ill'.

Natural emphasis in TCM

One of the most attractive features of this oriental and classical body of medicine is that it emphasises natural and safe forms of therapy that do not carry with them any harmful side-effects or consequences. They do not have to accept the Western opinion that they have to first get worse before they can get better. In the hands of a properly trained professional, TCM cannot possibly damage a person's health or diminish their well-being since no one needs to be forced to fit in with a therapy that is not entirely suited to his or her natural needs and requirements. All TCM therapies work essentially with and not against the body's own natural functionings.

Patient choice in TCM

Patients attending for treatment at a TCM surgery will be able to avail of a surprisingly wide and varied selection of treatment options. Indeed it will commonly be the case that a combination of different therapies of a specifically Chinese character will be used together. In a real sense it is this ability and knowledge to thus combine a number of possible therapies that is the distinguishing mark of the fully professional practitioner of TCM as contrasted, let us say, to the Acupuncturist who is restricted to the use of more severely limited treatment options.

It is the claim that TCM, taken as a whole and entire system of medicine, not just as one isolated branch or other, can treat any ailment a human being is heir to, whether it be predominantly physical, emotional, psychological or spiritual in character. In this sense, TCM is holistic by definition.

Prevention and health in TCM

Before going on to explain the wide variety of branches or components of TCM as a whole in some detail it is useful to briefly highlight the fact that it is concerned first and foremost with prevention of illness. Its pre-eminent wish is to avoid all forms of sickness. Its aim is to so strengthen and reinforce the individuals' existing health that he or she will not succumb to illness in the first place.

Indeed as knowledge of its health-enriching potential spreads, more and more people are approaching TCM to enhance, enlarge or perfect their health. Therefore, in direct contrast to Western medicine, it is not only sick or unhealthy people who can benefit from this multi-faceted, ancient and profound form of medicine.

Caution

A word of caution is appropriate at this point. It is because TCM is so wide ranging in its therapeutic options and effects that prospective patients must be aware that its mastery requires several years of dedicated and painstaking study. There are no short-cuts to competence in TCM. Only fully qualified practitioners, who consequently belong to established professional bodies, which offer full Professional Indemnity and Public Liability Insurance, along with demanding compliance to a recognised Code of Ethics and Practice, should be entrusted with the rare and precious commodity of one's health care.

To be absolutely sure of any practitioner of medicine every patient should consult the appropriate professional body to ensure practitioner competence and malpractice insurance cover.

The Therapies of TCM

Moxibustion

In China there is no separate word for Acupuncture. The Chinese terms *Zhen Jiu* are equivalent to *Acupuncture-moxibustion*. So closely are the two related that they cannot be spoken separately in Chinese. Although *Moxibustion* is a word that derives from a Japanese rather than a Chinese vocabulary it is an entirely Chinese form of therapy that uses heat. Instead of using acupuncture needles to pierce through the skin, a special herbal substance called *Ai Ye* (artemisia sinensis) is used to produce a mild and very gentle form of heat over the acupuncture point or injured body surface area. The herbal substance has the marvellous property of sending heat deeply into the tissue and muscles of the affected part and quickly brings relief in complaints as widely diverse as recent bruises or longterm painful joints.

Moxa forms

Moxa, which looks like a khaki coloured cotton wool, can be clinically used in a variety of ways, the following being the most common:

Moxa punk The moxa wool is shaped by the practitioner into tiny cones before being placed over an acupuncture point. As it slowly and gently smoulders, sending heat deep into the point area, the patient experiences a calming sense of warmth and comfort. When the heat builds up gradually to the verge of discomfort, the moxa is removed by the practitioner. During the course of a single session many cones might be used on a variety of different points.

Large cones Larger moxa cones can be used on top of a bed of herbal substances placed on the patient's skin so that as the heat is transmitted to the patient's body it picks up some of the herb's medicinal property on the way through the herb bed. A widely used herb in this type of moxa therapy is raw ginger, called *Sheng Jiang* in Chinese, which is sliced into a piece roughly the size and thickness of a 50p coin. By placing the moxa cone on top of the herb its warming effects are both boosted and concentrated.

Moxa Roll This resembles a large cigarette and is used to heat up wider areas of the body. It can be used in the Clinic but also given to the patient to take home for self-treatment. This particular type of moxa is extremely popular in China and the Far East, with every oriental 'medicine chest' containing several such rolls.

Moxa Uses

Moxibustion has an extremely extensive treatment range, including virtually any type of recent (sport) injury, fall, bruise, blow, twist, sprain (e.g. ankle) or stiffness (e.g. frozen shoulder, elbow, neck). It is also extensively used to treat a number of menstrual problems as well as different forms of joint, back, and muscular pain, even of long standing nature. It is used in the treatment of many pathological conditions that have coldness as an essential ingredient of their make-up.

Massage

In Chinese this therapy is called *Tui Na* which means 'pull and grasp' but involves a great deal more. Quite unlike any form of Western massage it is seen as a specific part of medicine. It is used to treat disease, not to simply promote relaxation or dispel muscular tension.

The techniques used are so extensive and varied that medics in China have to specialise in this therapy alone since there is not enough time to devote to other medical modalities. A strong physique is essential, as are many hours of relentless practice to gain proficiency. If one does not have the requisite strength to begin with one must first build up a powerful body before even starting to train in this branch of medicine.

A wide range of illnesses are amenable to Chinese Tui Na therapy. For example, a whole area is dedicated to the treatment of very small children, who the Chinese call 'milk babies', to correct digestive and bowel disorders commonly encountered in such infant patients. Indeed parents can be taught some of the simpler techniques to use on their offspring at home.

Quite remarkable success stories have emerged from China with regard to the spectacular results achieved by Tui Na in the treatment of Polio and other types of paralysis. Although the prospective Chinese patient can choose between Acupuncture and Tui Na, it would be a mistake to assume that it is preferable because less painful in adult use. Nothing could be further from the truth since the insertion of acupuncture needles, by an expert, is entirely painless, while Tui Na, because it must of necessity penetrate to levels deep within the patient's body, can be distinctly uncomfortable. Many Tui Na specialists in China are blind.

Qi Gong

This is a therapeutic spectrum of exercises taught to patients by their TCM practitioner, to be performed repeatedly for up to several hours daily. These essentially physical exercises which can concentrate on the patient's use and control of breathing are often combined with more meditative practices, and can be performed in any position, even lying in bed. The persistence and dedication with which these exercises are practised even by severely sick and debilitated patients frequently surprises Western observers.

The Qi Gong exercises are simple in themselves but their results can be remarkable. Such healing exercises are viewed strictly as medical treatment and are expected to achieve results in diseases as varied as defective lungs, heart, liver or kidneys, poor circulation, weak digestion and the like, to very profound life-threatening ailments like a stroke or even cancer.

In China, Qi Gong, which means 'repeated work on the vital energy', has entire hospital departments given over to it. Some Qi Gong master practitioners develop astounding powers whereby they can treat and even move their patient's body at a distance of several feet without any physical contact. The best of these practitioners are famous throughout China and are regarded as highly valuable medical experts.

Tai Ji Quan (T'ai Chi Ch'uan)

This is a more generalised form of exercise and meditative therapy which is not exclusively medical in application. It is often used, nevertheless, as part of the extensive 'treasure house' of TCM to strengthen and invigorate the entire person, either to assist in recovery from illness or, alternatively, to build up resistance to future attacks or health breakdowns. It has been graphically described as 'the subtlest form of Acupuncture' and within its own sphere of expertise it can effectively not only promote healing but so boost the immune system that the person becomes increasingly resilient and therefore resistant to infection and disease. In this latter fashion it could be seen as a workable form of real 'health insurance'.

Many TCM practitioners practice either Qi Gong or Tai Chi, or both, precisely to ensure such preventative benefits. An unhealthy practitioner, in any form of medicine, is a poor advertisement, and should be avoided on the grounds of common sense alone. It should be mentioned that although many people teach Tai Ji in Europe the skill and knowledge of this practice is variable in the extreme. As a rule of thumb, an unhealthy practitioner is not a useful teacher.

Cupping Therapy

This medical modality is not confined exclusively to TCM. It has counterparts in other systems of medicine. It involves the use of vacuumised suction cups placed on the skin over an acupuncture point or injured part of the patient's body. The main application of what was historically called 'Horn treatment' is the rapid alleviation of injury or pain related ailments. A secondary use is reserved for the treatment of more chronic complaints. It can be effective too in the treatment of the Common Cold.

Cupping therapy can be very easily combined in one treatment session with both Acupuncture-Moxibustion and Tui Na therapy, although, of course it can be used alone. The size and number of suction cups used in any session will be determined by the location and severity of the complaint. This treatment is not painful or distressing in any sense, although the vacuumised skin area can sport a purplish-blue circular discoloration for a few hours, or even a few days, after treatment. Because of this it is rarely if ever used on apart of the body that is visible to public inspection.

Die da ke

This is a much more restricted and specialised form of TCM therapy than any we have looked at so far since it concerns itself almost exclusively with the treatment of various types of injury or physical damage to the body, traditionally assumed to be acquired during the course of some war-like pursuit or in martial art training.

Literally the terms translate as 'Hit and Fall Therapy'. Renowned Kung Fu masters and monks from the Shao Lin temple recorded several hundreds of different treatment procedures to cope with the complex multitude of injuries and hurts encountered in such a setting.

It is mentioned here because although it selectively uses every other branch of TCM in its own therapy it is just beginning to surface in the West as a specialised area of study and possible use.

Nutritional therapy

This is called 'Food Medicine' in Chinese and actually uses food, either in its use or elimination, as a specific form of medical treatment. It has nothing to so with diets as we know them in the West. Second to Herbal Medicine(which we will look at in a moment) the knowledge of food therapy in TCM is extensive. It involves knowing precisely how different foods, food types, medically affect not only the physical body but also and equally the mind, feelings and indeed whole personality of the patient. Not only the type of food but also its method of selection, preparation and consumption are explained in the greatest detail by the practitioner.

It is safe to say that the majority of patients consulting a TCM practitioner will be given individually-tailored instructions regarding their food and drink intake throughout the duration of their treatment period. Nutritional therapy is such a basic and essential form of TCM that ignorance of its application would exclude a person from being regarded as an authentic TCM practitioner.

Therapeutic Counselling
As previously noted, TCM is ideally preventative in outlook and operation. Its aim is to prevent an ailment rather than letting it develop to the stage where it must be medically treated. Therapeutic Counselling in TCM explains the ways that illness may be prevented.

The TCM practitioner goes deeply into the reasons why the patient is presently sick but does not stop there. A thorough examination is made of the factors within the individual's life-style, that made the illness likely to occur in the first place. All patients attending TCM clinics will receive extensive instructions about how they should modify their living habits not only to recover more quickly from their present ailment but also to avoid its recurrence, or something similarly related, in the future. Health education is part of every visit to the TCM clinic.

Therapeutic Counselling is such an indispensable aspect of all TCM, that no matter what treatment option is employed, it cannot be omitted from any session. In a sense it is the most radical and traditional of all forms of TCM therapy. The ability of the practitioner to offer this option will distinguish the amateur from the true professional.

Herbal Medicine
This branch of TCM is the most extensive and widely used in China. When a Chinese person wishes to distinguish the medicine of his country from, say, Western Medicine he refers

to the former as Zhong Yao 'Chinese Herbal Medicine'. Although other branches of TCM may presently be better known and practised in the West, Chinese Herbal Medicine is the heart of TCM. A professional practitioner of TCM who had no knowledge of herbal medicine would be a contradiction in terms to the Chinese. A very famous doctor, Dr. Sun Si-miao, of the sixth century summed up this point by noting:

'Those practitioners who use either Acupuncture or Moxibustion alone are not brilliant physicians. This is especially true of those who use Acupuncture-Moxibustion or Herbal medicine in isolation. A proper practitioner of Chinese Medicine uses Acupuncture and Herbal Medicine together'.[1]

The range, variety and complexity, intricacy and applications of Chinese herbal medicine would require an entire book, or series of books to describe adequately. There are, for instance, well in excess of 60,000 substances used in hundreds of prescriptions. Prescriptions are dispensed traditionally in the form of raw herbs, treated herbs, patent herbs. pills, lozenges, tablets. powders, tinctures, teas, infusions, decoctions, ointments, balms, salves, oils, lotions, plasters, poultices, sprays, rubs and indeed every other type of medical preparation conceivable. The Clinical effectiveness of Chinese herbal medicine is greater in many instances than Western drug therapy and has the added advantage of being free of harmful side-effects.

So effective, extensive and safe is Chinese herbal medicine that a western researcher has concluded: 'China can claim to have the most ancient and sophisticated medical system in the world'.[2] A description such as that cannot easily be ignored.

1 *Chen's History of Chinese Medical Science* by Hsu and Preacher. Oriental Healing Arts Institute, Los Angeles, U.S.A. 1977 p.49
2 *Handbook of Complementary Medicine* by Stephen Fulder. 1984.

Acupuncture

by Tom Shanahan, M.A. (Oxon.), C.Ac.(Nanjing)

Seven hundred years after Marco Polo's journey to China, President Nixon's tour in the 1970s pulled aside the 'bamboo curtain' to reveal to the western world some of the secrets concealed for thousands of years by the ancient civilisation of the Middle Kingdom.

One of the most exciting and beneficial of these revelations was the treasure house of Chinese medicine in general and Chinese Acupuncture in particular.

Up until that time Acupuncture had been known to only a very small number of people in the West. Since then, interest has spread like wildfire. Patients have sought practitioners and newly emerging practitioners have been looking for training in ever increasing numbers. At the present time 'Acupuncture is one of the most popular and effective contemporary healing techniques, practised in almost every country on the globe' (*The Natural Family Doctor* by Dr. Andrew Stanway. Century Books, London, 1987 p.268).

What is Acupuncture?

Acupuncture, as the book just noted explains, 'is part of a comprehensive medical system that has survived over millennia'. It involves the insertion of extremely fine, pre-sterilized, stainless steel needles at predetermined points on the body surface to restore internal health. Put simply, the purpose of inserting Acupuncture needles is to release blockages and stimulate the correct flow of *Qi* (pronounced 'chee') throughout the body. Qi is the body's vital energy — it keeps the blood circulating, warms the body and fights disease.

Historical Origins of Acupuncture

Acupuncture is the main form of medical treatment received by over half of the world's population, used in conjunction with other forms of TCM and boasts extremely old origins. For example, a rudimentary form of Acupuncture, suggested by the archaeological discovery of stone needles (literally 'bian shi') has been dated to the New Stone Age period — 8,000 to 5,000 B.C. Its literary heritage extends back over 2,000 years to the Han Dynasty, 206 B.C. to 220 A.D., which is still conceived of as the 'Golden Age' of Chinese medical literature. The Han Dynasty is universally renowned for providing the 'bible' of Chinese Medicine, namely, *The Huang Di Nei Jing* (The Yellow Emperor's Compendium of Internal Medicine) along with *The Nan Jing* (The Classic of Difficulties) and many other seminal texts. This classical medical literature still supplies the primary resources of modern-day Acupuncture theory, and is in use in medical teaching colleges throughout China and indeed the world. 'China can claim to have the most ancient and sophisticated medical system in the world' (*Handbook of Complementary Medicine* by Stephen Fulder, 1984).

The Theory behind the Medicine

The philosophy or wisdom that lies at the root of all TCM, and indeed some other forms of oriental healing, is based upon a notion of wholeness, appropriateness and proportion. It maintains that these three ingredients are essential for health and that the absence or even lack of any of them will result in ill health. It is just this that explains *Yin* and *Yang*.

This philosophy however, does not ever see the person in total isolation from their surroundings. On the contrary, in diagnosing a patient, (i.e. a person who has lost some of the essentials just mentioned) it takes into serious account the whole life style and total environment of the person, including not only past history, day-to-day work and relationships, mental, emotional, intellectual physical, social and spiritual functionings, but also the geography and climate of where they live. All these factors are examined because it is believed that the human individual is one elementary component of the world, not something radically different to it and as such all human beings depend for their well-being upon factors such as those just noted. Put slightly differently, an imbalance, disruption or deficiency in any of these factors could well result in sickness.

The most fundamental belief is that the body knows how to keep itself healthy and will do so naturally unless it is hindered or thrown off balance.

The state of balance necessary for all healthy living depends on a careful avoidance of extremes. The middle way and not the extremes is where health is found. The Chinese describe this avoidance of all extremes, this embracing of the middle way, as the 'harmonisation of Yin and Yang'. These two terms are used to denote opposite but interconnected ends of a continuum which, in health, is in a ceaseless state of flux. Yin and Yang are merely at opposite sides of the spectrum.

They depend upon each other, support each other, both draw upon and feed from each other, but most importantly balance each other out so as to avoid all extremes. This is what is meant by *wholeness*. There is never too little or too much; neither deficiency or excess. This is what is meant by *appropriateness*. The individual is as they should be in the prevailing situation; they are in harmony with and at ease in their surroundings. As the ancient book of *Qoheleth* states: 'There is a time for every purpose under Heaven'. The constant but everchanging interbalancing of Yin and Yang ensures that precisely the right thing happens at the right time. This too explains what is meant by proportion. All disease comes from lack of harmony between Yin and Yang.

The deepest desire of this philosophy is to ensure that Yin and Yang are always harmonious so that disease cannot arise and that health grows in abundance and quality. The medicine of the East, unlike that of the West, is based firmly and pre-eminently upon a central notion of health and well-being rather than upon sickness and disease. This is the greatest point of contrast between the two and provides the insight into why they are so vastly different.

A very simple example can be used to highlight the essential point. If the body becomes too hot (a relatively Yang, excess, condition) or too cold (a Yin condition) then the body's own endeavours will be to restore equilibrium by, in the first instance, cooling down (e.g. by producing sweat) or, in the second, by warming up (e.g. by shivering which involves rapid movements, which in turn encourages the build up of body heat).

It is only when the body cannot, for whatever reason, successfully and thoroughly achieve this re-balancing and re-harmonisation that the orientally-trained doctor steps in to assist the ailing body. The aim is always and only to assist the body to put itself right. It never contradicts or confuses the body. It lends a hand only when needed and only for as long as is needed.

The ideal of oriental medicine, so easy to explain but not always so easy to quickly achieve, is to preserve, strengthen and enlarge a person's health so that they will not succumb to illness or disease but instead will enjoy life to ever-increasing fullness.

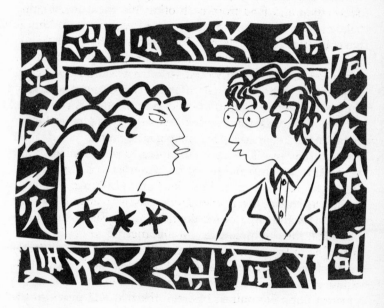

Diagnosis

Diagnosis lies at the very heart of all Chinese medicine. The physician, before treating, must discern precisely what is amiss in the patient. The means of doing so are vast and extend over millennia into the antiquity of oriental medicine. Two of the major diagnostic methods rely upon examination of the tongue and pulse of the patient. So important are these two examinations that they have been regarded as the foundation stones upon which all Chinese medical diagnosis rests.

Both are immensely complex, intricate and difficult to master. Their mastery demands endless time, effort and knowledge, but repays all expenditure by offering extensive, clear and reliable insight into the causes of ill health in the patient.

We can briefly outline some of their different features. First, with regard to the tongue, diagnostic information can be obtained by visual markings, swellings, indents, cracks, hollows, protrusions, moisture, one then looks at coating colours and thickness, concentration of coating in a particular tongue area, or its complete absence. We then turn to the tongue's size, deviation to left or right, upcurl or downcurl, movements sideways, its length, width and breadth. This examination gives the skilled and experienced practitioner a detailed and penetrating picture of the presenting pattern of disharmony or disease. Even different areas of the tongue can be examined to gain information about different parts of the body or even different aspects of the patient's personality. Not even the underside of the tongue is neglected.

Secondly, with reference to the pulse, there are nine distinct pulse palpation areas on each of the patient's wrists which are always felt by the three fingers of the physician pressing together to three different depths on each wrist. Traditionally there are twenty-eight pulse 'qualities' or characteristic pulse configurations which can be distinguished by skilled palpation to discover the precise nature and extent of ill health. The information on offer is proportionate only to the knowledge and expertise of the practitioner.

No traditionally-trained oriental medic would ever forego or neglect to avail of the treasure house of diagnostic information made available exclusively by recourse to these two fundamental diagnostic methods. Constant use of both could indeed be regarded as the authenticating mark of the true professional practitioner of any branch of Chinese Medicine.

What Acupuncture treats

Acupuncture treats people who complain of a deficiency or

break down in their health. It can also be used to enhance and boost the health of an already healthy person so that they do not become prone to illness or attack. It can focus on physical, psychological, emotional or even spiritual disorders with equal effect. Indeed, because Qi, Yin and Yang do not differentiate between the physical, psychological, emotional and spiritual, it can be said that Acupuncture always treats the patient on all of these levels. In Acupuncture as in all forms of TCM in full the treatment is tailored to fit the patient and not the disease. While much current research into Acupuncture is 'specificist' in its orientation — i.e., it attempts to identify particular Acupuncture points for particular complaints in the same way that Western medicine deploys specific drugs for specific complaints — it is traditional to treat each patient wholly and individually.

The type of Acupuncture treatment used will depend on the following:

— The nature of the complaint itself. Some complaints are by their very nature more severe or serious than others. This will determine the extent and type of treatment prescribed.
— The length of time the complaint has been there will also have some bearing. Generally speaking, more recent disorders are more easily and rapidly eliminated than those which have been present for a number of years. Acupuncture, however, can be equally helpful in both chronic (long lasting) and acute (coming sharply to crisis, not chronic) conditions.
— The frequency and type of TCM treatment administered can determine the likely outcome of therapy.
— The skill and experience of the practitioner cannot be discounted. Nor can the general state of health and well-being of the patient be disregarded in determining the effectiveness and speed of Acupuncture treatment.

What happens between treatments and how well the patient keeps to the instructions of the practitioner can also influence the speed of recovery, or otherwise. There is no limitation in terms of age, sex or condition regarding Acupuncture treatment. The very young or extremely old can be treated and pregnant women can be greatly assisted also.

Visiting the Acupuncturist

The first consultation can last anything between thirty and sixty minutes, or more in cases of complex medical histories. A very detailed medical history is taken and patients currently on a course of drugs should bring them along at the first visit. Even when a complaint has already been diagnosed by another practitioner, the Acupuncturist will perform an Acupuncture diagnosis using the methods described above and taking into account the patient's total environment and life-style as also outlined above.

Once the diagnosis has been made the patient's skin is swabbed with a bactericidal solution prior to the painless insertion of the Acupuncture needles. The patient may either remain seated or lie on the treatment couch throughout the session. A small number of needles, say three or four, are quickly inserted, most commonly somewhere between elbow and fingertips or knee and toe tips. Points on the back or chest can also be used — indeed Acupuncture points can be found on almost every part of the body. It may be necessary to undress or to partially undress.

The needles are then manipulated to ensure a characteristic sensation, in the local area or radiating some distance from it, of heaviness, distension, pins and needles, slight numbness, tingling, warmth or coolness. These sensations are a necessary aspect of treatment and in some cases can be fairly intense. It is simply not true to say that one 'feels nothing' — if one feels nothing it is because nothing is happening! The needles are left in position for twenty minutes, or for a shorter time for infants or children.

Patients are often very pleasantly surprised at how calming, soothing and relaxing the treatment can be and some even fall asleep. Already sleeping babies have been known not to awaken even when the needles are inserted. Acupuncture needles, by marked contrast to every other type of needle, are of a hair-like fineness, and it is this that allows such insertions to go virtually unnoticed.

When the Acupuncturist removes the needles he/she reminds the patient of the medical advice given during the session. This may pertain to diet, life-style, exercise, or may include herbal or other remedies to be taken. The client is then encouraged to take things easy for thirty minutes or so, to allow the treatment to 'settle'.

Subsequent sessions will last from twenty minutes (the typical length of time in China) up to an hour. Practitioners usually see patients once a week or once a fortnight. Acupuncturists may attend to more than one patient at the same time, in separate rooms. In this case, the patient will be asked to relax while the Acupuncture needles remain in place. The practitioner will be available at the end of the session to answer any questions.

Clinical Safety and Sterile Procedure

All Acupuncture needles are used exclusively upon one patient at a time. No possibility of cross-infection by using the same needle on two or more patients is permitted by any serious Code of Practice. All Acupuncture needles are pre-sterilized by recognised Agencies and some General Hospitals which specialise in such sterile procedures, which are carried out by Autoclave or other methods approved by the Department of Health.

Some Acupuncturists use only disposable needles, and if you are concerned on this score, you should ask which safety procedure is employed by the practitioner and to see the Acupuncturist's Certificate of Autoclave Sterilisation. Common sense would also dictate that the surgery itself is clean, tidy, well lit, well aired and in such a condition as to encourage the patient's confidence.

Practitioner Training

Professional practitioners of Acupuncture are concerned by the fact that patients sometimes say that they have 'tried Acupuncture before and it didn't work'. What emerges, on further discussion, is that the practitioner they have previously attended was not properly trained — he or she fell far short of being a fully- trained professional.

Acupuncture is a comprehensive medical system which is extremely valuable in the hands of a professionally trained practitioner. Before embarking on any course of treatment, however, the patient should be sure that the Acupuncturist has undertaken a minimum of intensive training.

Professional medical training in China begins with three years general medical and diagnostic studies, including clinical experience, after which the student specialises in one area of medicine, continuing to study and work in in that area — acupuncture, Chinese herbalism, massage, etc. The training should also include one whole year spent as a supervised trainee-practitioner in an established Clinic. This aspect of medical training cannot be safely omitted or shortened. All prospective patients, therefore, must make it a priority to raise the question of Clinical training with their practitioner since the very safety and effectiveness of any subsequent treatment could well depend upon its adequacy.

All Clinical training should preferably be carried out under the expert guidance of a Clinical Supervisor trained in China and experienced in working in the largest teaching hospitals.

Because Traditional Chinese Medicine in general, and Acupuncture in particular, is such an extremely demanding form of medical practice it necessitates years of concentrated and exclusive study to master. Because this is the case the public should be wary of any practitioner who claims to offer Acupuncture and a hotchpotch of other combined therapies, such as Homeopathy, Osteopathy, Chiropractic, Physio-therapy, Naturopathy, Massage, Reflexology, Western Medicine, and so on. This does imply that a practitioner can under no circumstances combine methods of treatment, but were this the case, it is necessary to be fully trained in Acupuncture regardless of previous qualifications. Traditional Chinese Medicine is a comprehensive medical system with a philosophy, theory and practice of both diagnosis and treatment.

There is a myth that Alternative and Complementary Medicines will not cause any harm, or do not have side-effects even if improperly administered. This is not the case — even Reflexology, one of the gentlest forms of Natural medicines is contraindicated in some cases.

Editor's note: Acupuncturists listed on the following pages are members of professional acupuncturists' associations. They are listed by Association and a description of the professional standards required for membership is given for each Association. As has been stated in the Introduction, it is also advisable to check out a practitioner's reputation and his/her success rate among patients.

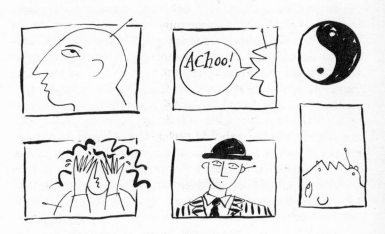

Practitioner Insurance

Practitioners listed below belong to professional associations which assure them of both Professional Indemnity and Public Liability Insurance, or carry such insurance individually.

Research:

It may be of particular interest to medically qualified readers to note the following sources of information about research into the effectiveness of Acupuncture. In the past four years, over 400 studies have been carried out in Britain alone, comparing and evaluating different aspects of Chinese and Western Medicine. The nature, scope, variety and results of these researches can be examined by consulting the *Index Medicus* or instigating a computer search programme on *Medline*. Some of the more recent Chinese research has been published in English under the heading: *The Second Symposium on Acupuncture and Moxibustion and Acupuncture Anaesthesia*. This volume alone contains over 640 abstracts from research projects presented at the 1985 conference in China. A companion volume entitled *Selections from Article Abstracts on Acupuncture and Moxibustion*, selected from over 900 recent research papers presented at the First World Conference in November 1987 in Beijing, includes 568 abstracts in a huge 712 page work.

Five Element Acupuncture

by Celine Leonard

Celine Leonard *trained at the College of Traditional Chinese Acupuncture in Leamington Spa. She then spent 2 years doing further training in her field while maintaining a private practice, and returned to Dublin in October 1989. She now works at Turning Point in Dublin, at Iomlanu in Dundalk and from her own clinic.*

The introduction of the ancient Chinese medical system to the West has been an important element in the birth, growth and development of holistic and complementary medicine. This article will reflect on that process and on the adaptation of the Chinese model of diagnosis and treatment to the particular needs of Western Culture. It will also give an explanation of the model of Chinese Medicine popularly known as *Five Element Acupuncture*, (more recently called *Leamington Acupuncture* in view of its location in England). I hope to show that whereas Chinese Medicine gives us access to an immense body of classical theory and practical knowledge, it is crucial that we neither simply transplant a system of medicine from a totally different culture nor reduce it to an adjunct to our own Western Medicine, but actively participate in the process of adapting it to the particular needs of post-industrial Western society.

This process means understanding not only the needs of Western individuals, but knowing also how the cultural framework of Chinese society has shaped the tradition recently made available to the West, as a coherent body of knowledge and practice which comes from the Chinese classics that is as integrated to the needs of the Western individual as it has been in the past to the needs of other East-Asian societies. This is an ongoing process and is happening as practitioners from different backgrounds seek to exchange models of theory and practice. I believe that Five Element Acupuncture has been part of the beginning of that process since it originates directly from an understanding of the Chinese Classics, yet is based as a body of teaching, geographically and culturally, in the West.

51

The system of diagnosis and treatment which comes under the aegis of Chinese Medicine has never been monolithic. From the beginnings of ancient history, there have been schools which have striven to develop a coherent philosophy and medical practice from a philosophical understanding of the life process based on the mutually opposing yet complementary forces of *Yin* and *Yang*. Theories of diagnosis and treatment have risen and fallen from prominence throughout that vast history, at times attaining great popularity and influence and at others, relapsing into relative obscurity. Medical theory and practice had to adapt to particular cultural needs, ranging from the series of great epidemics that swept China to the vast differences in needs produced by the class system of imperial culture within China itself. Similarly, as Chinese medical theory spread beyond the boundaries of its country of origin into other cultures, it was gradually adapted to the needs of that particular host country. In effect this meant that the Chinese classics were absorbed and developed into an autonomous system adapted to the particular cultural needs of such countries as Japan, Tibet and Vietnam.

What we have available to us now in the West is a more precise understanding of how each culture's medical system is as particular to it as its customs, traditions and social forms. This understanding of the particular cultural bias of health and illness has been termed the 'clinical gaze' of any particular culture. This term seeks to describe the way in which the very definitions of health and illness are actually radically different in different cultures. Our Western model of diagnosis and treatment is firmly rooted in the history and preconceptions of Western culture, dependent on the cultural revolutions of the seventeenth century and the birth of the scientific method. Our legacy is a medical establishment which seems limited by its very specialisation as it divides the human subject between the fields of the body (physiological processes) and the mind (psychological processes), with the uneasily vague term of psychosomatic complaints as the link between them. It leaves us as consumers of a vast range of pharmaceutical products which are designed to restore the normal physiological processes or mental/emotional states.

The great strength of Chinese medicine is that it sees the human subject as indivisible and, like any other holistic discipline, rejects the dualistic separation of mind and body. What it has at its disposal is an extremely ancient and sophisticated system for understanding the energetics' behind and beneath both physiological processes and mental and emotional states — an energetics which unites them as an integrated whole. It also possesses the knowledge of how and where to intervene in order to restore the harmonious operation of the entire system so as to begin the process whereby the individual begins to experience a well-being that is more than the simple absence of symptom. This understanding of the actual energetics of the body distinguishes, for instance, acupuncture from a therapy like homoeopathy:

> 'Homoeopathy acts by amplifying in a subtle way a defence reaction of the organism, whereas acupuncture, like Chinese pharmacology, aims more to strengthen the natural mechanisms of the vital force within an individual than to fortify the body's defences.'[1]

Chinese Medicine has a unique map of the human body, based on its understanding of the energetics of the human system, and sees it as expressing the same laws that operate in the natural world at the same time as it exists in a social world. This map of the body's energy pathways, uniting organs and pathways into an integrated whole, has been perfected over thousands of years and exists alongside a sophisticated diagnostic system for understanding the root cause of various symptoms.

Chinese Medicine is also unique in the way in which it understands the place of the human being in the larger sphere of our natural world. Unlike dominant Western ideology, it does not separate the human individual from the natural world, but sees human life as an unique expression of the same energies which operate on a vast scale in the processes of the universe and in the familiar scale of the human as a creative and social creature, subject to harm from both natural and social forces.

---

1   Survey of Traditional Chinese Medicine, Claude Larre and Jean Schatz, p. 104

It is also more important to realise, however, that a medicine must be tailored to the particular circumstances of the people it seeks to serve. Ted Kaptchuk has shown how the very nature of Chinese culture means that the individual's sense of self as well as her/his experience of distress is radically different from that of individuals in the West. Chinese culture binds the individual much more closely to family and social groups than that of the West, lacking as it does our cultural history of individualism and the particular problems of alienation and separation that causes the individual in Western culture. Furthermore, although Chinese medicine embraces the connection between physical and psychological realities, patients and practitioners alike, it emphasises the physical at the expense of the psychological/emotional and mental.

'The methodology (of Chinese Medicine) has always taken into account the psychosomatic truth that psychological and physiological processes are interactive and have a shared clinical significance . . . as emotional and physical concomitants of a single Yin-Yang experience. Nevertheless, contemporary Eastern and Western people tend to experience different ends of this continuum in their lives . . . The sense of self, purpose and meaning in life is fundamentally different. The contemporary Western patient tends to experience selfhood as individual centred and monitors his changing state in intensely personal terms, while the contemporary Chinese patient tends to view selfhood as situation centred and illness and health in physical terms' [2]

Furthermore, as Kaptchuk points out, the cultural frameworks of illness and well-being 'not only influences the clinical care but also has a great impact on medical theory and the formalised voice of medicine' [3] Western individuals are more openly preoccupied by existential issues which enter into their expectation of health care.

'Family relationships, work and career issues, life style management, sexual problems and stress reduction are all part of a Western patient's health concern... For many Westerners, the non bodily aspects of their beings are at times more accurate indicators of their health problems, constitutional configurations and Yin-Yang balance.' [4]

2   Journal of Chinese Medicine, Number 24, p.8-9
3   Ibid. p.10

What Kaptchuk points out is that, whereas the original classics of Chinese medicine openly discuss the emotional and existential aspects of an individual's being, historical and cultural pressures have systemically deleted such dimensions from recent text book presentations of Chinese Medicine, favouring a much more physiologically biased approach. The tradition which would include consideration of the emotional/psychological/spiritual aspects of human life has been preserved outside the formalised teaching, particularly since the Chinese revolution brought the ideological concerns of the revolution to bear on the practice and systematised presentation of the tradition of Chinese medicine.

In the model of diagnosis known as Five Element Acupuncture, or Leamington Acupuncture, each human being is seen as a unique creature embodying the larger forces which operate in the universe. The natural world is seen as an expression of the operation of those basic forces and energies which are familiar (indeed overfamiliar) to us in the process of the seasons, the yearly cycle of birth, growth, maturity/harvest and decline. Behind or within this familiar cycle are the energies and forces which each find particular expression in particular seasons. The theory represents an elaboration or unfolding of the theory of Yin/Yang into seasonal dynamics, and an understanding that every human being expresses in physical, mental and emotional ways, the same forces/energies which operate in the universe.

These forces are termed *Elements* or *Phases* in order to avoid the Western idea of static rather than dynamic forces. They are named as the elements *Wood, Fire, Earth, Metal* and *Water*. The element *Wood* is seen as operating most fully in the process of germination and growth which has its greatest expression in Spring. The element *Fire* is seen as having its greatest expression in Summer and in the process of ripening brought about by warmth. The element *Earth* is seen as primary in the late Summer, the pivot of the year, and in the process of the maturity brought about by late ripening which creates the harvest. The element *Metal* is seen as represented in the season of Autumn and in the simultaneous process of

4. Ibid.

harvest and decline. The element *Water* is seen as most fully represented or embodied by the season of Winter and in the process of recuperation, rest and renewal that is the necessary precondition for the rebirth of Spring.

In the Five Element model of diagnosis and treatment, the human being is seen as representing in a smaller scale and in a unique way the same basic impulses of creation. This is the point where it differs most radically from the orthodox Western perspective which sees each individual as a composite of a body maintained by the operation of physiological systems such as the cardiovascular, renal, hepatic, etc., and an autonomous sphere of psychological and mental/emotional process which becomes the domain of different practitioners. Five Element Acupuncture sees the human subject as embodying and expressing the elements in such a way that they operate indivisibly on the physical, mental and emotional levels.

Although one cannot equate Western and Chinese physiology, Five Element Acupuncture shares a basic map of the body in terms of a cooperative community of organ-systems. Each element is seen as represented in the body not only by linked organ-systems, but as the expression of the Element in physical, mental and emotional process. So the Element *Fire* is represented on a physical level by the Heart and the Cardiovascular system. But it is also represented by the unique capacity of each and any individual to express and provide warmth, intimacy, communication and community in their lives and in those around them. This extends the operation and meaning of the Element Fire into all those areas which we have culturally and figuratively associated with the Heart.

The Element *Earth* is expressed or represented in the person by the stomach and the spleen; organs involved in the transportation and transformation of the nourishment taken into the body for its sustenance. However, an understanding of the expression and operation of the Element Earth within any individual extends into the whole area of nourishment and to the relationship of the Self to Other. If the Element Earth is strong and healthy within an individual, she/he will not only be adequately nourished physically, but also able to nourish others and accept nourishment in the form of support and caring — to feel at home and grounded in the world.

The Element *Metal* is represented in the body by the organ systems of the lungs and the colon, and the physiological process of exchanging/creating waste, but its meaning and operation extends into the realms of worth and self-respect; that is the capacity of each individual to appreciate his/her own individual worth, quality and individual 'preciousness' and that of others around.

The Element *Water* is represented in the body most obviously by the organs of the Kidneys and Bladder and the mechanisms involved in the metabolism of water. But the meaning and operation of the Element Water extends beyond physiology into the realm of the conservation and storing of life processes. It is the element that 'pushes the organism to the actualisation of all its potentialities' — and thus its meaning and expression extends into the realm of survival, will, ambition and intention, skill and cleverness.

The Element *Wood* is represented in the body by the organs of the liver and the gallbladder. Whereas in the Western world of physiology, the fundamental role of the organs is restricted to metabolism, as represented by the Five Elements Model, the Element is instrumental in the organisation of the bodily process and of mental processes so that the energy of the Element is represented in human creativity and planning, decisions and judgements. Just as the Element Wood is the force represented in the essentially orderly and ordered process of creativity and growth, so the balanced Wood energy within an individual extends into areas of structuring, orderly and balanced planning, judgement with its basis in inner vision.

Although the description of the Five Element model is necessarily metaphoric in that it explains the operation of the Element within the human mind and psyche, the system is mapped precisely on/in the body in terms of the relationship between the organ systems of the body and the under-standing of energy pathways and acupuncture points. Similarly, each element has a precise set of associations in colour or hue of the face, sound or intonation of the voice, emotion, and odour as well as the greater associations of the seasons. In health and well-being each and every element will be invisible since its operation and expression in body, mind and emotion is absolutely appropriate. However, when an individual comes under stress and begins to express that stress in terms of symptoms; physical, mental or emotional, the elements will become visible precisely because they are not operating properly and appropriately.

So in health and well being, any individual expresses freely and appropriately the impulses and energies categorised in the elements — giving and receiving warmth and intimacy appropriately, nourishing and able to accept nourishment/support appropriately, confident in their self-worth and that of others, able to conserve energy and express their potentiality, creating appropriate structures of thought, planning and organisation. In the community of the body, each element nourishes and controls another so the physical, mental and emotional process operates smoothly and the individual expresses harmony and well-being.

However, given that human beings come under climatic and environmental stresses and can express those stresses in symptoms, Five Element diagnosis holds that in each individual there will be one particular element which will operate as a *Causative Factor* of distress in the individual. Established at an early age, it is seen as operating as a weak link in the community of the body and the true source of the various symptoms which can arise in any of the other organ systems. Furthermore, since Five Element Acupuncture sees the operation of the elements not just as operating in physiological terms, it would understand that imbalance in the body will manifest in behavioural terms and will be expressed primarily in the inappropriate expression of that one element, so that a person can express the weakness of their Causative Factor not just as a physical symptom, but also in terms of an energetic imbalance in the expression of that element. So the Causative Factor is as likely to be expressed as an essential, fundamental lack of joy or nourishment, self-worth, appropriate structure, as in any physical symptoms which points to the malfunction of any particular organ system.

The system of diagnosis in Leamington Acupuncture

revolves around the establishment by the practitioner of which Element and its attendant organ-system is operating as the Causative Factor of distress. This is done not only by detailed attention to the nature of the symptoms but also by attention to the predominant colour, odour, vocal intonation, emotion and behaviour, tongue and the pulses which indicate the condition of each organ and the relative balance of the whole. This overall pattern will indicate which of the Elements/ organ systems needs support and what support, whether building or quieting, and warming with moxa in addition to needles if appropriate.

Treatment is the process of re-establishing balance, through the insertion of fine stainless steel needles into acupuncture points, either stimulating or sedating the energy of a particular organ-system. The initial diagnosis with a Leamington practitioner will last approximately one and a half hours as the practitioner gathers detailed information about the nature of the symptoms being experienced and about the overall situation of that person. Treatment thereafter is generally once a week for about 45 minutes, and then as improvement happens, becomes less frequent. The speed of improvement varies more according to the person than the label of the complaint. Some people are much improved after one visit, others require more extensive treatment. The actual process of treatment is that it provides the necessary support so that the person can begin the process of recuperation. As they gain in strength, they no longer need that support in the same way so that the practitioner becomes in effect redundant.

Leamington Acupuncture holds that consistent and appropriate treatment of the Causative Factor will produce changes of a much wider/deeper range than the mere removal of symptoms. With support to the Causative Factor, strain is lifted from all the other organ systems so that the body begins the process of regaining and maintaining equilibrium. This type of change includes the fact that the client will express herself/himself as feeling better in themselves, as experiencing the relief of widely varied and seemingly unconnected symptoms, and of finding an improvement in their capacity not just to cope with the circumstances of life but to live a more satisfying life as they express the qualities of the elements in more balanced and appropriate ways.

The process of adaptation of the ancient system of Chinese medicine to the concerns of Western culture has already been happening. However, in order to make this process easier, it is important that we understand the particular demands of our own culture and the way in which cultural influences impinge on our well being. Similarly, we cannot be dismissive of those forms of therapy which have grown up in the West in answer to our cultural needs here. In my own practice I have found that at times a combination of psychotherapy and acupuncture can be particularly effective in integrating changes in a person's life. Just so, we must be careful not to reduce a person to a collection of symptoms or a life-style which needs to be adjusted, but to be aware of how genuinely unique each individual's experience is as she/he comes into contact with the social structure of gender, class and race. The theory of Chinese medicine offers us a wonderful model for helping the process of restoring well-being to an individual. As it takes its place among predominantly Western therapies its true value and potential will be clearer precisely because it has had to adapt to such different circumstances and to people who have never heard of Tao, Yin, or Yang and yet want to experience wholeness and well-being in their lives.

Listing of Practitioners of Acupuncture and TCM

Practitioners who provided this information state that their fees range from £10 concessionary fee to £30 non-concessionary fee for first-time visits. £20 for first-time visits and £15 for subsequent visits are the usual fees.

Practitioners of Traditional Acupuncture

Practitioners trained at the College of Traditional Chinese Medicine at Leamington Spa in England are represented as a professional body by the *Traditional Acupuncture Society*. The TAS requires members, before joining, to have achieved a comprehensive understanding of the theory of acupuncture and to have demonstrated clinical competence. Members must also have passed examinations in Western Medical

Sciences. The Society also provides Professional Indemnity and Public Liability for its members. All members are bound by the Society's Code of Ethics and by a Code of Practice which includes stringent standards of hygiene and sterilisation for equipment and needles. The TAS produces a leaflet which acts as a good introduction to anyone thinking of having acupuncture.

TAS Members in Ireland are as follows :
Celine Leonard, Tel. 01-542140 for details of private clinic; also Turning Point, 2, Landsdowne Gardens, Shelbourne Road, Ballsbridge, Dublin 4. Tel. 01-602600/680588; also Iomlanu, 36, Castle Rd., Dundalk. Tel. 042-32804 (Mondays).

Listings of Acupuncturists and Acupuncture associations

The Professional Register of Traditional Chinese Medicine(PRTCM)

The PRTCM is the associated professional body of the Irish College of Traditional Chinese Medicine (ICTCM), which offers a three year intensive course in Acupuncture and the other forms of TCM outlined in a separate section on TCM (see p. 00). The ICTCM enjoys close links with the Nanjing College of TCM and ICTCM graduates are invited to attend post-graduate intensive clinical training courses there. Several students have already availed of this facility and future visits are presently in preparation. The ICTCM also enjoys close links with the Chengdu College of TCM since it is the mother college of the two resident Chinese doctors who teach at the ICTCM. Specially devised Clinical post-graduate training courses are being planned for PRTCM members for 1990. Practitioners of TCM who pass an examination set and supervised by the Council of the PRTCM, as well as graduates of the ICTCM are eligible for membership.

Members, all of whom practice the whole range of TCM and not solely Acupuncture, are covered by full and international Professional Indemnity and Public Liability Insurance underwritten by Lloyds of London and are bound by a Code of Ethics and a Code of Practice.

The PRTCM is '. . . dedicated to the development of the highest standards of medical training and practice to ensure the firm establishment and growth of TCM in Ireland (and)it regulates the professional conduct and ethical behaviour of its members.'

The Register circulates a Directory of practitioners to interested parties, such as conventional medical practitioners, hospitals, health centres, training institutes and other health care bodies and also sponsors the following publications: *Code of Ethics*; *Code of Practice*; *Acupuncture information pamphlet*; *Insurance cover pamphlet*; *Acupuncture* an information booklet for *The ICTCM Syllabus*; A quarterly Newsletter *SHENMEM*.

The PRTCM and ICTCM were founded six years ago by Thomas J. Shanahan, M.A.(Oxon), C.Ac.(Nanjing) China. Further information about the ICTCM and PRTCM is available from: The Secretary, 100 Marlborough Rd., Donnybrook, Dublin 4. Tel.01-603313/978906, and from The Registrar, 1 Hunsdon Rd., Iffley, Oxford, England. Tel. Oxford 772560. The PRTCM is a founder organisation of the Institute of Alternative Medicine (IAM) described in the Introduction. It is also a founder of the Irish Acupuncture Council (IAC).

PRTCM Members : Ireland and Overseas

Cork:
Birgid Posthuma, 72, Summerhill, St. Luke's, Cork. Tel. 021-504484
Dublin:
Sylvia Bradshaw, 65, Hollybrook Rd., Clontarf, Dublin 3. Tel. 01-331976; Christopher Davala, 12 St. Mary's Rd., Ballsbridge, Dublin 4. Tel. 01-689731; Tony Hughes, 1, Leopardstown Drive, Stillorgan, Co. Dublin. Tel. 01-880352; Mary Plunkett, 100 Marlborough Road, Dublin 4; Liz Rackard, 17, Leinster Road West, Rathmines, Dublin 6. Tel. 01-978906; Tom Shanahan, The Marlborough Clinic, 100, Marlborough Road, Dublin 4. Tel. 01-603313/978906; Vincent Sex, St. Anne's Square, Portmarnock, Co. Dublin. Tel. 01-460520
Galway:
Assumpta Roache, Knockatee East, Dunmore, Co. Galway. Tel. 093-3885; Thomas J. Shanahan, Acupuncture Clinic, The Crescent, Galway. Tel. 091-55389
Kildare:
Monica Teahan, Ballysax Rd., Mooretown, Kilcullen, Co. Kildare. Tel. 045-81398
Limerick:
Marion Fenton, (Clinic) 8, The Crescent, Limerick. Tel.061-310166; (Home)

"Doonass", Clonlara, Co. Clare. Tel. 061-354111; Reg. sick children's Nurse, Reg. General Nurse, Reg. Midwife.
Mayo:
Maggie Deffely, Glenisland, Castlebar, Co. Mayo. Tel. 094-22940
Sligo:
Christopher Davala, Sligo City, Tel. 071-85298
Wexford:
Gerry Morrissey, Connagh, Fethard-on-Sea, Wexford. Tel. 051-97368

1990 Graduates

Donegal:
Dolores McCullagh, Quay Road, Dungloe, Co. Donegal. Tel. 075-21129
Dublin:
Arlene Capot, "Dundarave", Woodside, Sandyford, Co. Dublin. Tel. 01-943803; Neil Kelly, 20, Leopardstown Grove, Foxrock, Dublin 18. Tel. 01-945254; Ann Mary Luttrell, 12, Kingsland Park Ave., S.C.R., Dublin 8. Tel. 01-604745; Doreen McGouran, 8, Ballsbridge Avenue, Dublin 4. Tel. 01-601856
Galway:
Pat Curran, 14, Rahylin Glebe, Ballybane, Co. Galway. Tel. 091-53471; Geraldine Flannery, Convent of Mercy, Tuam, Co. Galway. Tel. 091-48031; Eileen Leahy, 28, Glenina Heights, Galway. Tel. 091-55389
Kildare:
Jim Burns, Newbridge Road, Naas, Co. Kildare. Tel. 045-76041
Laois:
John Freeman, Mary Street, Durrow, Co. Laois. Tel. 0502-36125.
Limerick:
Celine Casey, 8, Cambridge Close, College Court, Castletroy, Limerick. Tel. 061-330149
Waterford:
Kevin Power, Garrycloyne, Colligan, Dungarvan, Co. Waterford. Tel. 058-68279

PRTCM Practitioners Overseas

Jonathan Bruce, Tel. Oxford 778448
Sue Davies, Gwynedd, N. Wales, Tel. 0492-581507
Francois de Menthon, Cambridge, Tel. 0223-358121
Richard Druitt, Combe, Oxon., Tel. 0993-898106
Bridget Henderson, Oxford, Tel. Oxford 249706
Ted J. Kaptchuk, Cambridge, Mass. U.S.A. Tel. 354 1744
Ronald McDonald, London SE 25 Tel. 653 2541
Tom Shanahan, Oxford, Tel. Oxford 772560
Richard Temple, London NW 11 Tel. 455 3743
Geoffrey Wadlow, London SE 5 Tel. 701 7107

The Association of Irish Acupuncturists (AIA)

The AIA is a professional Acupuncturists association which includes Acupuncturists who have trained and qualified in diverse training centres and countries. It was formed to promote Acupuncture and to maintain professional standards among Acupuncturists.

Its members carry Professional Indemnity and Public Liability Insurance and are bound by a Code of Ethics and Practice. A Teaching School affiliated to the AIA has begun and is in the first stage of acceptance by the Acupuncture teaching hospital in Beijing. The AIA publishes a Newsletter for its members and interested parties. Further information about the AIA is available from Tony McGinley, 9, Westcourt, Tralee, Co. Kerry. Tel. 066-24694 Further information about the School is available from Marie Gallagher, "Suncourt". Leafdale, The Lough, Cork. Tel. 021-964470. The AIA is a founder organisation of the IAM, described in the Introduction.

AIA Members

Cork:
Teresa Connolly, Paddock, Drinagh, Co. Cork. Tel. 028-30314; Kees van Dam, Gregane House, Roscarbery, Co. Cork. Tel. 023-48110; Carmencita Chemont Dekkers, Reenroe, Drimoleague, Co. Cork. Tel. 028-31364; also, 5, Sydney Place, Cork. Tel. 021-31364; Clinical Psychologist: Dr. Martin Dekkers, Reenroe, Drimoleague, Co. Cork. Tel. 028-31364; also, 5, Sydney Place, Cork. Tel. 021-506077; Medical Homeopath: Betsy Diddierens, Princes House, Castletownsend, Co. Cork. Tel. 028-36381; Gary Murphy, 62, Summertown Road, Wilton, Cork. Tel. 021-42559; John (Kerry) Murphy, 62, Summertown Road, Wilton, Cork. Tel. 021-42559; Babs O'Byrne, Riverside House, Townsend Street, Skibbereen, Co. Cork. Tel. 028-21101; Noel O'Reagan, Arnica House, 8, Langford Row, Cork. Tel. 021-964470; Elma Von Royen, Carrigmore, Waterfall, Bantry, Co. Cork. Tel. 027-70004; Oswald Schmidt, 52, Earlwood Estate, Cork. Tel. 021-962268
Dublin:
Dr. Josephine Freeney, 5, Lakelands Drive, Stillorgan, Co. Dublin. Tel. 01-888174; Joy Lennon, 25, Chalfont Park, Malahide, Co. Dublin. Tel. 01-451258 (afternoons); John McLoughlin, Natural Health Clinic, 55, Ranelagh, Dublin 6. Tel. 01-757132; Annette Tallon, 6, Martello Terrace, Sandycove, Co. Dublin. Tel. 01-842294
Galway:
Linda Heffernan, 67, Tirellan Heights, Galway. Tel. 091-69676; Rea O'Beara, 69, Mayola Park, Newcastle, Galway. Tel. 091-24093; Eilin Ni Riordain, 38, Upper Abbeygate Street, Galway. Tel. 091-67416; Bruce Du Ve, 38, Upper Abbeygate Street, Galway. Tel. 091-67416
Kerry:
Fiona Maxwell, Main Street, Castleisland, Co. Kerry; Tony McGinley, 9, Westcourt, Tralee, Co. Kerry. Tel. 066-24694
Limerick:
Sam Kingston, "Pinaroo" South Circular Road, Limerick. Tel. 061-28002; John O'Mahony, 22, Upper Mallow Street, Limerick. Tel. 061-27265
Tipperary:
Halogue Malone, Mount Falcon. Borrisocane, Co. Tipperary.

Fees charged by AIA Members vary from £10 concessionary fee to £25 non-concessionary fee for a first-time visit. £15 to £20 is the most frequently charged fee.

The Acupuncture Foundation of Ireland (AFI)

Further information about the AFI is available from 87, North Circular Road, Dublin 7. Tel. 01-387699/388196

AFI Members

Athlone:
Mr. Bruce Du Ve, Athlone appointments, Tel. 0902-78750

Cork:
Pierce Hennessy, Lr. Windmill Hill, Youghal, Co. Cork. Tel. 024-93519/024-92754; Dr. Ray Shanker, c/o Gregane House, Roscarbery, Co. Cork. Tel. 023-48110

Dublin:
Carmel Bradley, 138, Philipsburg Ave., Fairview, Dublin 3. Tel. 01-370543; Adam Bux, Apollo Buildings, Dundrum Rd., Dundrum, Dublin 16. Tel. 01-988127; Elaine Glynn, 37, Hainault Drive, Cornelscourt, Dublin 18. Tel. 01-895446 (evenings); Michael Gygax, 201, Ashcroft, Raheny, Dublin 5. Tel. 01-387699; David Howett, 10, Offington Court, Sutton, Dublin 13.Tel. 01-387699; Mrs. P. Kelly, 25, Ailesbury Road, Ballsbridge, Dublin 4. Tel. 01-696436; Carmel McHenry, Wellington Place, Dublin 4. Tel. 01-387699; Dr. M.S.Khan, 123 South Circular Road, Dublin 8. Tel. 01-534854; Deirdre Phelan, 12, River Gardens, Glasnevin, Dublin 11.Tel. 387699; Nick Power, 51, Lower Albert Rd., Glenageary, Co. Dublin.Tel. 01-387699; Dr. Adnan Rabie, Sundis Health and Beauty Salon, Main St., Blanchardstown, Dublin 15. Tel. 01-216116; Stephen Shaw, 6, Monkstown Grove, Monkstown, Co. Dublin. Tel. 01-804821; Noeleen Slattery, The Belgrave Medical Centre, Belgrave Square, Dublin 6. Tel. 01-975666; also, Rathcoole, Co. Dublin. Tel. 01-589672; Leo Trayner, 218, Whitecliff, Rathfarnham, Dublin 16. Tel. 01-941534; Ronald Turner, "Cluain Ard", Stillorgan Road, Blackrock, Co. Dublin. Tel. 01-884327; James Walsh, 111, Walkinstown Road, Dublin 12. Tel. 01-508232/ 534854; Tony Walsh, 87, North Circular Road, Dublin 7. Tel. 01-388196; Alison Larkin, Finglas West, Dublin 11. Tel. 01-387699

Galway:
Alan Brannelly, 1, McDara Road, Shantalla, Galway. Tel. 091-22631; Nora O'Connell, 18, Mary St., Galway. Tel. 091-66482 (after 5pm); Bruce Du Ve, 38, Abbeygate Street, Galway. Tel. 091-67416

Limerick:
Frances Lynch, Fern Hill House, Eyon, Cappamore, Co. Limerick. Tel. 061-381317

Leitrim:
Saskia de Jong, Drumkeeran, Co. Leitrim. Tel. 01-387699 (enquiries)

Meath:
Gemma Dillon, Dromrone House, Nobber, Co. Meath. Tel. 046-52360

Offaly:
Derry O'Malley, 13, Healy Street, Tullamore, Co. Offaly. Tel. 0506-41600

Wicklow:
Catherine English, 59, Herbert Park, Bray, Co. Wicklow. Tel. 01-387699

The Irish Register for Traditional Chinese Medicine (IRTCM)

Dublin:

Ann Campbell, 54, Kennelsfort Road, Palmerston, Dublin 20. Tel. 01-262349; Eileen Dowley, 147, Rathfarnham Road, Dublin 14. Tel. 01-905275; Patrick Flaherty, 108, Kimmage Road, Dublin 12. Tel. 01-518388; Dr. Michael Maguire, 31, Hazelwood Court, Artane, Dublin 5. Tel. 01-471444; Ann Marie Mollereau, 20, Palmerston Park, Rathmines, Dublin 6. Tel.01-973223

Kildare:

Peg Cronly, Main St., Clane, Co. Kildare. Tel. 045-68015

Kilkenny:

Ann Marie Mollereau, Kilkenny (Mondays). Tel. 01-973223 (appointments)

Independent Practitioners

Dublin:

Michael Cawley, Centre Point, The Village, Cabinteely, Co. Dublin. Tel. 01-852831/01-692934 (Residence); Cert. in Advanced Acupuncture Studies from Beijing College of Chinese Medicine in China; Olive Gentleman, 2, Laurel Pk., New Rd., Clondalkin, Dublin 22. Tel. 01-592460 (also Reflexology); Dr. Catherine Larkin, 32, Upr. Baggot St., Dublin 4. Tel. 01-683996; M.B., member of the British Acupuncture Association, C. Ac., Nanjing; Practises TCM — Acupuncture, Moxibustion, Chinese Herbalism, Dietary Advice.; also at 1, Goldsmith Tce., Quinsboro Rd., Bray. Tel. 01-683996; also at the Dublin Well Woman Centre. Special interest in endometriosis, menstrual, pre-menstrual and menopausal problems; Dr. Anna Lee, 9, Lakelands Rd., Upr. Kilmacud, Stillorgan, Co. Dublin Tel. 01-885233; Dr. Ann O'Rourke, 30, Iona Crescent, Glasnevin, Dublin 9. Tel. 01-306438; also Counselling; Paula Smyth, 196, Upr. Rathmines Rd., Dublin 6. Tel. 01-961533

The Academy of Chinese Medicine offers part-time courses in Acupuncture for practising acupuncturists. Courses will commence in Autumn 1990. All classes will be instructed by Dr. Anna Lee, an acupuncture specialist from the Beijing College of Chinese Medicine. For further information write to: Secretary, Michael Cawley, The Academy of Chinese Medicine, 81, Merrion Rd., Dublin 4. Tel. 01-852831/885233

Northern Ireland:

Roisin Golding, The Gate Lodge, 1, Baldon Park, Belfast BT9 5LG. Tel. Belfast 664573; Dr. B. Gonsalves, 72, Maryville Park, Belfast BT9 6LQ Tel. Belfast 662729; Dr. James T.S. Lee, 1a, Galway Park, Dundonald, Belfast BT16 OAN. Tel. Dundonald 89644; Ralph McCutcheon, 150, High Street, Holywood, Co. Down. Tel. Holywood 5953; M.K. Sharkey, 106, Strand St., Derry BT48 7NR. Tel. 0504-261532

Shiatsu

I would like to thank Catherine Sutton for her help with this article.

Shiatsu is a Japanese healing art and has its roots in the same oriental tradition as acupuncture, moxibustion and oriental herbalism. The concept of Yin-Yang and the qualities of the Five Elements are the essential parts of Shiatsu treatment and diagnosis. These have been outlined in the previous articles on Traditional Chinese Medicine and Five Element Acupuncture to which the reader may refer.

In Shiatsu the basic premise is that the human being is a totality, is part of the life of the Universe and that energy creates and maintains life. This energy is known as *Ki* in Japan and as *Chi* in China. Ki circulates in the body along recognisable passageways known as meridians and gathers at points on the meridians which are known as tsubos. The word Shiatsu can be translated as finger or thumb pressure. The practitioner of Shiatsu, by applying pressure to another person's body, aims to balance and harmonise the Ki energy. Because Ki energy is the basis of the body, mind and spirit, all of these aspects are treated by Shiatsu.

In general, a Shiatsu treatment covers the whole body. A variety of techniques such as rocking, holding, and leaning are used in addition to applying pressure with the foot, elbow, finger, thumb and hand. Occasionally, the practitioner will work with only one part of the body, such as head and shoulders, and will concentrate on the meridians in that area that require particular attention, depending on the nature of the ailment.

Shiatsu is an important part of preventative healthcare and is also effective in the treatment of most illnesses. Most illnesses have both a physical and emotional cause and Shiatsu treatment is as effective for depression as it is for something as physically obvious as *abdominal cramps*. A Shiatsu therapist sees that physical, emotional and spiritual blockages and negativities all create dis-ease. Shiatsu is effective for the treatment of sinusitis, migraine, irritable bowel syndrome, ulcers, constipation, depression, hyper-activity, arthritis, rheumatism, gout, back pain. Many of these

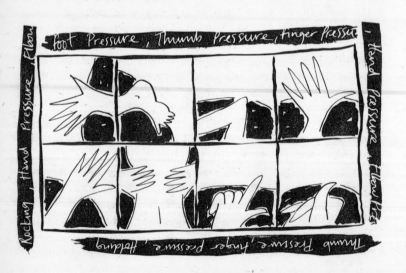

illnesses are stress-related so emphasis is put on looking at the cause of illness rather than just the symptoms.

The sensitivity of the practitioner to the energy of the person receiving Shiatsu is emphasised and Shiatsu is, in this way, most unlike Western medicine. Shiatsu massage will also heighten our sensitivity to our own bodies, teaching us to be aware of the signs that we are under stress, to relax and relieve tension.

Having a Shiatsu Massage

Shiatsu massage is a very special part of regular healthcare, and I will describe my own experience below. In this 'massage' the clothes are left on.

A Shiatsu massage begins with the feeling that practitioner and client are meeting with respect and empathy. The practitioner begins by 'centering' his or her own energy in order to work, and as this happens, one becomes aware of one's own energy. It is as if the calm, centredness of the practitioner mirrors one's own energy-state.

The massage itself begins with the client kneeling, usually using a low stool for support. As the practitioner's hands move over the body, identifying and easing into pressure on the tsubos, one can feel where one's energy is blocked, where there is resistance, and where the energy feels right. As the massage progresses, one's state of mind becomes more and more relaxed. The rush of random thoughts, worries, etc. slows down and one settles into a more meditative state of mind. There is just enough time to notice the grace with which the practitioner moves when it is time to lie on the floor-mat, and then the eyes close — at least mine do!

In general, we accumulate a lot of stress around the head, shoulders and back, and the work on these areas feels quite intense. There can be momentary pain as resistance in certain points eases, but any pain is soon followed by a sense of relief/release.

This sense of relief/release can be quite dramatic and lasting if the blockage is relatively minor and short-lived, but may require regular treatments where the condition is more deeply-rooted. From session to session, the points of blockage, where pain is felt when pressure is applied, can shift. Gradually, the flow of energy throughout the whole body is corrected. Often exercises, stretches and dietary changes are advised as 'homework' and help maintain a good flow of energy and feeling of well-being.

As the massage continues, there is an accumulating sense of free energy, the counterbalance of the accumulated tension one started with. It is not just that each 'bit' of the body feels better, looser, but that one's whole mood and energy level lifts, and there is a sense of completion when the whole body has been touched. (See also Massage by Judith Ashton, Chapter Six below).

Body Sense

In Shiatsu, there are two basic qualities of energy which can be recognised with practice, called *Kyo* and *Jitsu*. Yin-Yang refer more to the direction and tendency of energy, Kyo and Jitsu to the quality, degree and intensity. Kyo is where energy is deficient and there is a feeling of emptiness/tiredness or of being unsatisfied. Jitsu is where there is a fullness or excess of Ki and the feeling is of overactivity/tension. Jitsu arises out of Kyo; where there is deficient energy in one part of the body, an emphasis of energy, or Jitsu will develop in another part in order to balance the organism as a whole.

Where the imbalance is mild, Kyo and Jitsu will be imbalanced only in the meridians and in the person's overall energy. Where the imbalance is more serious, it will be evident in bodily organs and systems. Symptoms will vary according to the severity of the imbalance. Corresponding to Kyo and Jitsu, the techniques of manipulation to balance the energy are called tonification — those used to create stimulation, and sedation — those used to diminish energy. By exerting these influences the total body energy field is reorganised, creating balance.

Kyo and Jitsu apply not only to the energy within the body, but will also be reflected in the person's outer expression, self-description, emotions, intellect, preferences and attitude to life.

Energy

In a medical system whose philosophy is based on the concept of a unifying energy which takes various forms, it follows that our own body sense is important, reflecting the condition of our whole being. Thus sensations such as numbness, tingling, heat, cold, stiffness, pins and needles, in fact the whole range of body sensation has significance. In Western Medicine such sensations are treated as localised phenomena, or ignored unless causing actual discomfort. When discomfort does arise, it is treated locally and the organ or part of the body in question is viewed alone, separated from the rest of the body. The physical is separated from the emotional, the emotional from the spiritual, the human being from the environment, and so on. In Shiatsu, however, bodily sensations such as those above are taken as indications of the beginning or existence of imbalance. The *tsubos* and *meridians* on the outer surface of the body reflect the inner organs and systems as well as the emotional and spiritual state that the person is in. The practitioner will use his or her hands to create balance in the other person's energy field. An awareness of our own bodies can also help us to recognise the occurrence of imbalance and so we can take action so as to prevent serious illness from developing.

Such an awareness is, of course, gradually developed and is at odds with what we have been conditioned to think. For instance, in Shiatsu, the whole body is seen as a manifestation of energy and all illness as an imbalance in that energy. Although modern physics has discovered that there is an underlying unity between matter and energy, modern medicine still separates the physical from the emotional and spiritual. Analytic thought emphasises the difference between things, and our educational system is biased in this direction. The faculty of intuition, which is used alongside technical skills by the practitioner of Shiatsu, is denied its validity — but increasingly, many people are discovering for themselves the benefits of viewing the human being as a whole and of treating and preventing illness from that perspective.

Practitioner Training

There are two levels of training for Shiatsu — one is a quick 'do it yourself' style Shiatsu and the other is a training to use it professionally to treat ill people.

The 'do it yourself' Shiatsu can be learned in evening or morning classes over 8 — 10 weeks and these classes are available in various VECs, Adult Education Centres, Community Centres, various groups, etc. in Dublin and some other areas. Intensive training weekends are also offered to cover basic theory and techniques. The names of teachers are given below.

Professional training in Shiatsu is much more intensive and requires a greater commitment. While there is one school in Ireland offering such training there are also many schools in England, Europe and the USA, (not to mention Japan!). The School of Shiatsu and Natural Healing is offering a part-time residential Course over a period of a year. The Course commences in September and consists of five, nine-day programmes. A lot of study and practical work is necessary in between each programme. The Course will equip the participants to practice Shiatsu professionally. Further information is available from the Shiatsu Society of Ireland. (See below);

References:
Shiatsu Practitioners Manual by Saul Goodman. (Infitech Publications.)
Beginning Shiatsu by Elaine Liechti.(Unity Books.)

Listing of Practitioners

The Shiatsu Society of Ireland was formed in 1989 as an all-Ireland body to promote the use of Shiatsu as a healing art in itself and one which is compatible with virtually all other forms of treatment, whether orthodox or complementary. The Society also seeks to establish and regulate professional and ethical standards for the practise of Shiatsu in Ireland.

There are two levels of membership:
a) Practitioner, or full membership, which is open to those meeting the requirements set out in the Constitution and Code of Ethics.
b) Ordinary membership, which is open to all others, whether students or merely interested.

The following practitioners are available to give courses

and workshops at Community level throughout Ireland and are members of the Shiatsu Society of Ireland :

Anne Hyland, Tel. 066-58289;
Carmel Kelleher, Tel. 01-337735;
Josephine Lynch, Tel. 01-883378;
Joe McGuire, Tel. 01-484270;
Catherine Sutton, Tel. 01-966509.

Further information is available from : Joe McGuire, Secretary, The Shiatsu Society of Ireland, 12, Grange Park View, Raheny, Dublin 5. Tel. 01-484270

Shiatsu Society of Ireland Practitioners

Clare:
Mary Moran, Caherabona, Liscannor, Co. Clare. Tel. 065-81563
Cork:
Kerry Bradley, Farran, Mayfield, Bandon, Co. Cork; Seamus Connolly, 63 Westbury Estate, Wilton, Cork. Tel. 021-342794
Dublin:
Carmel Kelleher, Clontarf, Tel. 01-337735; Josephine Lynch, Mount Merrion, Tel. 01-883378; Joe McGuire, Raheny, Tel. 01-484270; Liam Murray, Dun Laoghaire, Tel. 01-842662; Also teaches T'ai Chi Qicong (Breathing exercises) and T'ai Chi Chuan (complete Cheng system); Mary Moran, Donnybrook, Tel. 01-602298; Also Reflexology; Catherine Sutton, Harolds Cross, Tel. 01-966509; Betty O'Toole, 6 St. Kevin Park, Dartry. Tel. 01-979762; Mary Walsh, Belgrove, Sandyford Village. Tel. 01-956883
Kerry:
Anne Hyland, Inch, Co. Kerry. Tel. 066-58189
see also Natural Living Centre, p.211
Louth:
Ann Finn, Dundalk, Tel. 042-77125
Northern Ireland:
John McKeever, 12 Gransha Ave., Belfast. Tel. 084-614495
Tipperary:
Joannes Barkery O'Brien, Ceol an Grá, Ardcroney, Nenagh, Co. Tipperary. Tel. 067-38172
Co. Wicklow:
Aisling Blackburn, c/o 29 Seacrest Bray, Co. Wicklow. Tel. 01-863000; Christiana Niels, Stewards Hse., Fort Granite, Baltinglass, Co. Wicklow. Tel. 0508-81559

Chapter Three

THE BODY'S FRAMEWORK

Osteopathy

I would like to thank Chris Campbell, D.O., for his help with this article, above and beyond the call of duty.

Osteopathy is one of the forms of healing that combines a western-scientific view of human anatomy and physiology with a philosophy that accepts that the body's Vital Force plays the major part in preventing and eliminating disease. It aims to stimulate the body's own healing mechanisms and systems by means of techniques of manipulation designed to restore the body's vitality, structure and function.

Andrew Taylor Still

The first school of Osteopathy was founded in 1892 in Kirksville, Missouri, U.S.A. by Dr. Andrew Taylor Still (1828 — 1917). Still was one of a settler family of Scottish origins, his father a physician and Methodist Minister. Influenced by a love of Nature and a keen awareness of the hardship endured by settler families, Still also trained in Medicine and practised among the settler or planter families.

Later, he was involved in the movement for the abolition of slavery and he served as a physician under Lincoln in the American Civil War from 1862 to 1864. In his practice and during the Civil War, Still began to feel that the current modes of medical practices were inadequate. This feeling grew and reached a climax when three of his own children died of spinal meningitis, despite the efforts of Still and his colleagues. In response, Still began independent studies, convinced that the remedy for disease lies in the body's own mechanisms and health-building systems. He focused these early studies on anatomy and physiology — the structure of the body, the nervous system and the circulation of the blood.

The Spirit of the Times

In Europe, at that time, Pasteur was gaining acclaim for his findings on micro-organisms, or germs, Lister was trying to introduce anti-septic surgical procedures ; there was a climate of discovery and of furious debate in the fields of biology and medicine. One of the most controversial debates was that between Pasteur and his colleague, Claude Bernarde. Pasteur argued that, for the purposes of understanding disease, the Organisms, or germs, should be studied, identified and controlled by the administration of drugs in vaccine or other forms. This theory, the *germ theory* of disease was established by Pasteur in 1864 and is still the dominant theory of disease in western medicine. Against Pasteur and the germ theory, Bernarde argued that the proper object of investigation was the human body, or the *Organism*. In the course of experimentation parallel to Pasteur's, another researcher, Bechamp, found that the organisms can only emerge and develop in a suitable environment, and by implication, that they often reflect a certain stage of illness, rather than causing it.

Famous Last Words

In Science as indeed in life, no debate is ever conclusively settled. This is borne out in relation to the germ theory by something Pasteur said in the company of friends and colleagues only hours before his death: 'Ah, Bernarde was right all along, it is the Organism'.

In Osteopathy, it is a maxim that 'There is no such thing as disease, only sick people'. Osteopaths do not deny that the germ theory is correct in some cases, but they prevent and treat illness by promoting the body's own systems.

Osteopathy in the U.S.

Osteopathy's roots are in western Medical Science, and in that context, it balances the emphasis (or over-emphasis) placed on drugs and germs by its big brother. In the US, Osteopathic

Physicians had been given equal recognition and rights to practice with other physicians in every State by 1973. There are now over 18,200 Osteopaths in North America, 14 Colleges of Osteopathy and Osteopathic Hospitals in most States. The American Osteopathic Association states that it:

'. . . seeks to provide that service (Osteopathy) as a separate and distinct medical group until such a time as the basic medical truths it proclaims become a part of the body and practice of contemporary medicine'. [1]

However, Osteopathy is more and more frequently practised in the US in conjunction with orthodox techniques and even drugs. Many now regard the UK as the place where Osteopathy is taught and practised with most regard for the original principles, even though its practice there is not as widespread as it is in the US.

What is Osteopathy?

Osteopathy is most widely known for the practice of manipulation of the bone structure. In fact Osteopathic adjustments to the bodily structure are designed not only to put bones in place but also to bring all parts of the body into structural harmony. One of Still's earliest stated principles is that 'The structure of the body is reciprocally related to its function'. Misalignment of the body's structure will affect the functioning of the organs and systems and dis-ease in any part of the body will be reflected in the structure. Osteopathic treatment aims to heal irritation or obstruction in the body's own curative systems. Osteopaths identify any abnormality by sight and by touch.

The musculoskeletal system is the framework on which the body rests (or aches, at times) and it also contains most of the pathways for the blood and neurological impulses. By restoring mechanical balance, these systems are freed from obstruction and the body's own healing systems can do their work. Diagnosis is also carried out by a concentrated and intense assessment of both the shape and the energy patterns of the body. For example, the way one holds ones head or

1 *Osteopathic Medicine; An American Reformation,* by George W. Northup, D.O.,F.A.A.O.(American Osteopathic Association, Ill., U.S.A.,1979)

shoulders, cold feet, limp or taut tissues, stiffness of joints etc. indicate not only the nature of a localised complaint, but also reflect the condition of the organs and mechanisms connected to that point. In examining the whole body, the Osteopath is concerned not to identify and name specific diseases, but instead, to assess the state of health of the patient as a whole person.

The Osteopathic Lesion

An area of abnormality identified by an Osteopath either by sight or by touch is known as a *lesion*.

A lesion can consist of
— misplaced structure;
— hardening of thickening in the soft tissues;
— alteration in the relation of one structure to another;
— change in the conditions of the cells.

The existence and location of lesions is indicated by:
— some abnormality in the position of the bones when at rest;
— some abnormality in the mobility of the joint;
— tenderness of the soft tissues over the prominences of the bone itself;
— some abnormality in the feeling of soft tissues;
— some abnormality in the feeling and appearance of the skin over the area of the lesion.

Lesions can be caused by:
— damage due to a fall, a bang, a twist, etc.;
— damage due to posture. This in turn may be caused by occupation, by a person habitually adopting a postural position that is off-balance, by an early injury or even by incorrect footwear. (See also The Alexander Technique;
— an injury to one area of the body can put stresses and strains on another joint where another, compensatory lesion can arise;
— a disease in one of the organs will be reflected in the musculoskeletal system. Each organ and each part of the body has a definable related part of the spine and it is on

the spine that this type of lesion, known as a reflex lesion, can be identified;

— an 'environmental' lesion is a lesion due to social, emotional, or other stress in the person's environment. The total environment of the patient is taken into account by an Osteopath, including relationships, housing conditions, psychological or emotional pressure due to work or other factors, etc.

Not all disease is caused by Osteopathic lesions, and this fact is recognised. However, a high proportion of disease is so caused, and can be cured by Osteopathic treatment.

Visiting an Osteopath

On the first visit, the Osteopath will carry out a thorough examination, for which it will be necessary to undress. A medical history will be taken, although Osteopathic lesions tell their own story. The initial examination can last up to 30 minutes, as can the subsequent treatment. Further visits will be shorter, from 10 to 30 minutes, depending on the type and extent of work needed. The treatment given is specific to the patient.

Length of treatment

Some conditions respond quickly to Osteopathic treatment, others take time. For instance, if there is stiffness or soreness following an accident of any kind this can generally be rectified in a few sessions. Persistent backache, or chronic conditions of most kinds will require treatment over a longer period. In the latter case, the practitioner of Osteopathy will give treatments designed to build up the body's strength before tackling an old lesion and its derivative problems. There is a myth of the Osteopath as a miracle worker, who straightens bent bodies at one fell swoop! The reality is that Osteopathy is addressed to the person's constitution, that manipulation can be overdone, and that there is no instant cure for weaknesses in the body that may have begun during childhood, or even at birth. Again, this varies with the individual but your Osteopath will indicate the duration of treatment required after the initial examination.

Reactions to treatment

The patient will be alleviated of pain as quickly as possible and remedial treatment for older lesions will follow. What is known as a *healing crisis* sometimes follows Osteopathic work on the body. The healing crisis is that part of any illness where the body is doing its utmost to expel the blockage, toxins or other factors causing dis-ease. For example, the healing crisis may take the form of an apparent 'ear infection',with the ear expelling toxins in the form of pus and the temperature rising above normal. It appears that the sickness has become worse, but a true healing crisis indicates that the worst is over, and that the person is getting better. Similar reactions to treatment from a Reflexologist are noted in the section on Reflexology.

An Osteopath will expect his or her work to be accompanied by good nursing, hygiene and a sensible diet, and will be available if a healing crisis does occur. The nursing techniques used in Osteopathy are Naturopathic, that is, they do not involve the use of drugs to suppress symptoms, instead a cold wrap, poultice, etc. will be used to assist the body in its work.

A healing crisis does not always follow Osteopathic work, this too depends on the individual. Where a healing crisis does occur, and is permitted to run its course, it has been my personal experience that the patient, on recovery, feels better than ever. Many people live with conditions of dis-ease, or average health, for a period of months or even years, feeling that at least it's not getting worse — however, nothing is static in nature, there is always either growth or decay. In Osteopathy, the gradual and related effects of the different types of lesions are recognised, dealt with and cured in accordance with the state of health of the individual and the bodily healing functions. Following a healing crisis, or when none occurs, Osteopathy is an enjoyable way of regaining health, each improvement is noticeable and builds on the previous step.

The treatment itself

Osteopathic treatment varies widely from person to person, and is therefore difficult to describe.

In contemporary times, physical, emotional and general environmental stress dictates that it is usually necessary for an Osteopaths to make adjustments to the back. In this case, the patient undresses, wholly or partially, and the Osteopath presses, rotates or pulls arms, shoulders, or vertebrae to make these adjustments. The Osteopath may work on the back itself, gently; the patient may lie on the back and clasp hands while the Osteopath presses on the shoulders to make an adjustment; the person may lie on one side first and then the other while the Osteopath makes adjustments to the hips. It is for this type of treatment, so commonly necessary these days, that Osteopathy has become known for clicks and immediate relief.

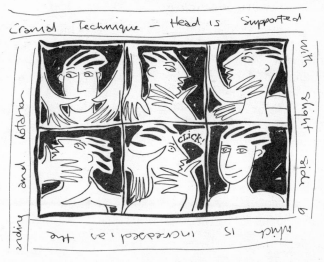

Where a person has suffered injury at birth, cranial massage (massage of the skull) is performed. Cranial injuries at birth may take the form of imperfect meeting of the skull over the fontennelle, or soft spot on a baby's head, imperfect conjunction of the neck and skull, or a variety of other forms. These in turn can affect the functioning of the brain to a greater or lesser degree by putting physical pressure or restrictions on a part or parts of the brain. Adjustments can be made to the skull and have been shown to be effective in treating serious under-development of the brain. In this kind of treatment by a skilled practitioner, both the emotional and the physical effects of birth trauma will be treated.

These are only two of a large number of Osteopathic techniques which may also include Reflexology. The unity of body, mind and spirit is assumed in Osteopathy and although it shares a view of Anatomy and Physiology with mainstream medicine, it also recognises *The Vital Force* and treats in order to allow it to flow freely and strongly.

'Man is triune when complete. First the material body, second the spiritual being, third a being of mind which is far superior to all vital motions and material forms, whose duty is to wisely manage this great engine of life.'
— Andrew Taylor Still.[2]

A New Era in Medicine

Osteopathy's social philosophy of Medicine is that the promotion of healthy life-styles is more desirable than the dominant ethic of identifying dis-ease and seeking to eliminate it through the administration of drugs to huge numbers of people.

One instance where Osteopathic technique has been combined with mainstream medicine to the benefit of all is the use of cardiac massage (massage of the heart) during heart operations or in cases of cardiac arrest. The aspiration that Osteopathic truths will be recognised by mainstream medicine has many obvious merits, particularly to those of us who have suffered chronic, 'minor' illnesses that simply cannot be treated by the ethic of 'repair, relieve or remove'.

References:
Introduction to Osteopathy. (The Maidstone Osteopathic Clinic, Maidstone, Kent.). *Principles of Osteopathy*. Edited and revised by John Wernham. (Published as above.)

Listing of Osteopaths

Irish Register of Osteopaths

Ireland has hitherto been unique in Europe in that no

---

2 *Philosophy of Osteopathy*, by Andrew Taylor Still. (A.T. Still, Kirksville, Mo., U.S.A. 1899, American Academy of Osteopathy, 1977.)

association existed to unify its practising Osteopaths. In 1989 a group of Osteopaths formed with the aim of creating a register of practising Osteopaths. This register will provide prospective patients and health professionals with a list of qualified Osteopaths practising in Ireland. Osteopaths on this register will hold a diploma of Osteopathy (D.O.), and will have completed a minimum of four to six years study at a recognised college. This will eliminate dubious practitioners and charlatans, protecting patients still further. The number of registered Osteopaths is expected to grow, fulfilling a public need for a natural, non-invasive and comprehensive osteopathic service. All members of the register may use the initials M.I.R.O. (member of the Irish Register of Osteopaths), after their name. The public may be thus assured thay are using a safe, experienced and completely trained Osteopath. The following list of Osteopaths has been supplied by the I.R.O. As the I.R.O. is a relatively new organisation, membership is still growing. An updated list is available from James Doyle or Gerry Flynn (see below).

Members of the Irish Register of Osteopaths

Cork:
Noel O'Connor, 36, Sheares St., Cork. Tel. 021-275456; Christopher Pardoe, 29, Castle Close Drive, Blarney, Co. Cork.
Tel. 021-381173
Down:
Ivan Bell, 89a Cranreigh, Hillsborough, Co. Down. Tel. 683390
Dublin:
Chris Campbell, 118 Cherryfield Rd., Walkinstown, Dublin 12. Tel. 01-501724; James Doyle, Garden Residence, 33, Wellington Place, Dublin 4. Tel. 01-606804; Gerry Flynn, 3, Merrion Court, Ailesbury Road, Dublin 4. Tel. 01-695525
Louth:
Philip Kearns, 46, Fair Street, Drogheda, Co. Louth. Tel. 041-31544
Tyrone:
Jim Myler, 4, Church St., Omagh, Co. Tyrone.

Chiropractic

by Joseph Gilmore, D.C.

Joseph Gilmore *is a Chiropractor and member of the Chiropractic Association of Ireland who practises in Dun Laoghaire in Dublin.*

Modern Chiropractic dates from 1895 when the first chiropractic adjustment was performed by Daniel David Palmer in Davenport, Iowa. Chiropractic is based on the fact that health maintenance and restoration are dependent upon the integrity and function of the nervous system. The nervous system controls directly or indirectly virtually all functions of the body. If the nervous system is interfered with by mechanical, chemical or emotional factors disease (dis-ease) will result. Chiropractors identify and remove this interference by conservative methods. Chiropractors, by choice, do not use drugs or surgery but in many cases will utilise nutritional and/or physical modalities such as heat, cold, galvanic or micro-electric stimulation, traction, etc.

The principles of modern Chiropractic have historical roots going back to about 400 B.C. and Hippocrates, the father of western medicine, said: 'In disease look well to the spine'. In the Eastern or Chinese tradition the roots of manipulation go back another four or five thousand years. In the United States of America there are approximately 30,000 licensed chiropractors. They are entitled by their education and the law to the title "doctor of Chiropractic" commonly seen as D.C.

Chiropractors recognised by the Chiropractic Association of Ireland have had a minimum of six years of university level study including internship and are now striving to gain legal recognition and to prevent the usage of the title "Chiropractor" or Chiropractic etc. by unqualified individuals.

The Doctor of Chiropractic considers the body as a total functioning unit. She or he gives special attention to the spine and the way it affects and is affected by the muscular, nervous, hormonal, circulatory, digestive and skeletal systems. The Doctor of Chiropractic relieves distress, pain and the noxious nerve impulses that cause many diseases by specific adjustments to specific vertebrae in specific directions.

Additional clinical measures may be used as indicated. When the nervous system is permitted to function optimally the natural healing processes of the body bring about the cure. The D.C. is especially known for successfully treating neuromuscular problems such as head, neck, arm and shoulder pain, mid or low back pain or sciatica. These are problems that affect most of us at one time or another and these are the reasons that most of our patients go to a chiropractor but actually the Doctor of Chiropractic does much more. Because of the pervasive scope and influence of the nervous system and the way it controls or regulates body function, interference or irritation can cause many and varied disturbances and diseases.

Many people visit the Doctor of Chiropractic for one problem and find their other problems improving or disappearing altogether. The same problem that is causing pain, irritation or malfunction in the mid-back for instance, may also be causing pain, irritation or malfunction in the stomach or small intestine. The same problem that is causing low back or sciatic pain may also be causing malfunction of the colon or reproductive organs. Women who have "monthly backache" along with other menstrual discomfort may find all symptoms improved when the spine is "put right". When the nervous system is free to express itself normally, healthfully, the body heals itself.

The modern chiropractor is trained to recognise problems that need non-chiropractic care and will refer to other specialists as indicated and will usually co-operate in providing multi-discipline care for those patients who need it. The Doctor of Chiropractic generally considers his 'care' as falling into one of three categories, i.e. *first aid, correction,* or *maintenance.* We will deal with each in turn.

Chiropractic *first aid* is the care necessary to help the patient over the acute stages of pain. Most patients go to their physician because they are in pain, they are hurting. The chiropractic makes the appropriate adjustment and the pain is reduced or eliminated. (Not all the pain goes away all at once all the time, I wish it did!) The chiropractor may also recommend ice, heat, ultrasound, etc. Now the patient feels better and may want to discontinue the care. The first aid phase is over.

Correction is that care that while starting with the first visit continues beyond first aid to eliminate the cause of the problems. In many ways the back can be compared to the teeth. Just because it is not aching today does not mean that there is no problem. Getting rid of the pain does not mean that we have fixed it, tooth or back. The post first aid care is necessary to reduce or eliminate the propensity, the chance of recurrence.

Maintenance care is the periodic care your chiropractor may recommend after you have reached a maximal level of health and stability from corrective care. Its aim is to help you stay in the best of health, at your peak. The chiropractor feels that you should take care of your body as you do your car. We may not be able to eliminate all problems in the future but we can avoid many of the more common ones. How often we see our chiropractor depends on the uses to which we put our body and whether those uses are appropriate to our physiognomy. We can't expect a person of sixty to be able to do the same work as he could at twenty or forty. We can't expect a woman of eight stone to carry or lift the same loads as a sixteen stone man.

List of Chiropractors

The Chiropractors listed below are members of the Chiropractic Association of Ireland (CAI) and the information was supplied by the CAI.

Cork:
Mark Cashley, D.C., Duntahane, Fermoy, Co. Cork. Tel. 025-32413; Billy Tague, D.C., Raleigh Lodge, Macroom, Co. Cork. Tel. 026-42116; Marie Murphy, D.C., Duntahane, Fermoy, Co. Cork. Tel. 025-32413
Dublin:
Gary Dennis, D.C., 126 Clontarf Rd., Dublin 3. Tel. 01-334026; Linda Finley, D.C., 5 Old Blakestown, Clonsilla, Dublin 15. Tel. 01-201362; Joseph Gilmore, D.C., 6, Charlemont Terrace, Dun Laoghaire, Co. Dubl.in. Tel. 01-800488; Owen Dennis, D.C., 126, Clontarf Rd., Clontarf, Dublin 3. Tel. 01-334026; Robert Finley, D.C., 107 Trees Rd., Mount Merrion, Co. Dublin. Tel. 01-882891; Lorraine Herricks, D.C., 126 Clontarf Rd., Clontarf, Dublin 3. Tel. 01-334026; Fionntan Mac Cuill, D.C., 14 Marrington Place, Dublin 2. Tel. 01-763686; Laurel Martin, D.C., 5 Old Blakestown, Clonsilla, Dublin 15. Tel. 01-

201363; Paul Noone, D.C., 2 Manor Heath, Marley Grange, Dublin 16. Tel. 01-946429.
Galway:
C. A. Gludworth, D.C., D.I.C.S., Roscam, Merlin Park, Galway. Tel. 091-51858; Jesse Lawrence, D.C., "Estelle", Tuam Rd., Galway. Tel. 091-55205.
Sligo:
Helga Wendt-Schmettau, D.C., Theur, Riverstown, Co. Sligo. Tel. 071-67686.
Northern Ireland:
Anne Matthews, B.Sc., D.C., Belfast Chiropractic Clinic, 228, Ormeau Rd., Belfast BT7. Tel. Belfast 641675/641015, Member of the British Chiropractic Asociation; Roy Hamley, D.C., as above.

Spinology

by Brigid McLoughlin

Brigid McLoughlin *is a practising spinologist based in Cork and a member of the Spinology Association of Ireland.*

Spinology is an art and practice which seeks to aid the well being of the individual by maintaining the integrity of the spine and nervous system. It was founded and established in 1979 by Reginald Gold. Mr. Gold was an eminent teacher and practitioner of Chiropractic for many years. With this background and his involvement in the Human Potential movement, combined with his interest in Eastern Mysticism he established America's first Spinal Tutorium in Philadelphia. He devised a concise and intensive course which places great emphasis on practical training ensuring that each Spinologist is totally competent and skilled when dealing with the spine.

The initial duration of the course is one year, after which the student Spinologist must establish a practice within the Spinal Tutorium. Here he or she is continually supervised and assessed while working on many people. When the student is seen to be proficient he or she is certified and ready to establish their own practice independently. The time period for certification differs for each Spinologist, but can vary from months to years.

The aim of Spinology is to allow each person to maximise their use of human potential by seeking to keep the body functioning at 100% of its genetic capacity. The chief director of all bodily function is the brain and its extension, the spinal cord which connects with the peripheral nervous-system of the whole body. To maintain chemical equilibrium and harmonise the balance within the body it is vitally important that there be no interference with the flow of energy through the spine.

Just as the brain is protected by solid bone (the cranium), so too is the spinal cord protected by bone which is segmented into twenty-four movable parts called vertebrae which enable us to twist and move with great flexibility. On either side of each vertebra there is a tiny hole through which passes a nerve trunk. The nerve trunks divide and subdivide to form the peripheral nervous system which connects with every part of the body. This whole nervous system therefore maintains communication between the brain and the body parts and vice versa.

So the vertebrae of the spinal column are designed to permit perfect movement and at the same protect the spinal cord. For the very reason that they are movable and flexible it is possible that some of these vertebrae become displaced out of their correct positions. When this occurs they interfere precisely with that which they are designed to protect. This interference is called *Spinal Obtrusion*.

When Spinal Obtrusion exists it hampers the free flow of nerve impulses to and from the body parts thus causing disequilibrium often malfunction within the body. Some examples of such malfunction are indigestion, migraine, constipation and lack of good physical co-ordination, emotional balance and self-healing ability. Spinal Obtrusion also results in impingement on the nerve trunks which can cause localised or referred pain and other related problems.

The majority of people who attend a Spinologist do so because of problems such as lower back-ache, leg pain, discomfort in the mid-thoracic area of the spine, or pain beneath the shoulder blades. Neck problems are also common and involve pain in the arms, across the tops of the shoulders, headaches, sensations of numbness or pins and needles.

Some examples of possible causes of Spinal Obtrusion are as follows: injury due to lifting, over-stretching, falling, car accidents, poor posture, severe tension or stress, certain occupations which necessitate the spine to be in an awkward position for long periods of time, childbirth, etc.

It is however, very wise to have one's spine checked without waiting until a problem occurs, as Spinal Obtrusion is often present without causing any awareness as such within the person concerned. In this way Spinology fulfils one of the roles for which it was originally intended; that is to be an effective means of body maintenance.

The Spinologist can detect Spinal Obtrusion by moving the fingers along the spine, thus 'reading' all the information given by muscle tensions, bone position, etc. This technique is called vertebraille. When an obtrusion is detected the Spinologist applies a gentle and precisely directed 'thrust' to assist the return of the vertebra to its correct position.

Some people attending a Spinologist may have quite severe and ongoing back problems. It is frequently necessary to have regular visits initially in such cases, and then periodic check-ups after that. Very often, attendant to a back problem there can be quite severe problems with the muscles and ligaments. In such cases the Spinologist may decide to do some deep massage to assist healing. It is sometimes helpful to combine Spinology with other complementary disciplines such as Acupuncture, Reflexology, or Relaxation techniques to name but a few.

When the spine is Spinal Obtrusion free, there is no interference with the nerve system, and thus the body's life-lines are open, allowing a free flow of nerve energy which in turn ensures the optimum function of the body. Periodic visits to a Spinologist will allow this to happen and hence the individual is afforded the possibility of functioning at maximum genetic potential.

Practitioners of Spinology

Cork:
Brigid McLoughlin, 1 Empress Pl., Summerhill North, Cork. Tel. 021-509075
Dublin:
Dermot Kelly, 46, Fortfield Park, Terenure, Dublin 6. Tel. 01-902565;
Stephen M. Shaw, 6, Monkstown Grove, Co. Dublin. Tel. 01-804821.
Galway:
Ray O'Beara, 44, Lr. Newcastle Rd., Galway. Tel. 091-24093.
Laois:
Patrick Kelly, New Road, Portlaoise, Co. Laois. Tel. 0502-22994.

The Alexander Technique

I would like to thank Frank Kennedy for his help with this article.

The Alexander Technique comes under the umbrella of health education rather than a treatment for illness.

Frederick Mathias Alexander was born in Tasmania, Australia, in 1869 and died in London in 1955. He was a Shakespearian actor, and he began to develop the Alexander Technique as a way to combat constant sore throats which led to voice loss and hoarseness. Finding that rest or medication brought only temporary relief, he came to the conclusion that it was something he was doing that was causing the problem.

Over a period of years, Alexander observed every aspect of his movements in front of a mirror. He discovered that he was pulling his head back when speaking, which led to sucking in his breath and depressing the larynx, thus increasing pressure on the vocal chords and resulting in hoarseness. He went on from this initial observation to study the interconnections of the whole body, finding that the head and neck position affect the chest, spine, pelvis and so on. He observed, further, that even when he thought he was moving his body correctly, he wasn't. Ways of moving and holding the body that felt comfortable and right were actually inhibiting the body's natural capacities and his sense of what was right was based on habit. Habit had become stronger than an instinctive sense of the body's natural poise. The Alexander Technique was developed as a means of re-educating this sense so that the body is fully and properly used, in a natural way.

The central principle of the Alexander Technique is that correct use promotes function, misuse inhibits function. Muscles, respiration, circulation, the nervous and lymphatic systems, joints and muscles are all affected by the ways in which we use our bodies. Mechanical defects in how we move and carry ourselves can impose wear and tear on bones and joints and many back problems are posture related. Correcting bad habits of this nature will ease related physical conditions such as asthma, rheumatism, headaches and fatigue.

Our sense of well-being, confidence, openness, is also enhanced by relearning our sense of natural poise and balance. Our emotions such as anxiety, anger, sorrow, fear, are all reflected in our body-language and in our bodily

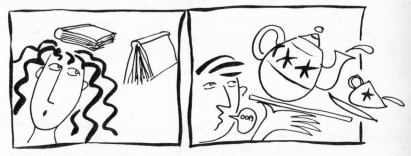

functions. When we overreact to situations, or when we experience fear, there are corresponding physiological patterns. The fright, or startled pattern is one example; it can become habitual that we react with this pattern to simple things such as someone calling us from behind. When this happens, our bodily functions are called on inappropriately. An underlying sense of anxiety may be at the root of such a pattern and anxiety can also be created in this way. By developing a sense of what is happening physically that is inappropriate and a sense of what is right, emotional and physical patterns can be unravelled and corrected. The Alexander Technique provides the opportunity to undo bad habits, to iron out the wrinkles in our responses and functioning in everyday situations and thus it enhances the body's functions and our emotional balance. It is both a preventive and a corrective method and it is a maxim that a degree of change or improvement is always possible.

The technique is taught to clients individually by trained teachers. Teachers of the Alexander Technique train full-time for three years. The number of lessons required varies, generally between 15 and 30 half-hour sessions. During the lessons, the teacher will gently move and guide the parts of the body into their natural and correct positions, instructing the student how to move from right position to right position. It is taught in the context of the student's daily regimen and does not involve exercises to be done at a special time. Instead, it teaches correct movement in our normal daily activities and the gradual reacquisition of our sense of natural balance. It encourages movement in a free and uninhibited way, with a sense of poise. It is not artificial, does not encourage rigidity and is tailored to the needs of the individual student. It is a joy to re-experience the ease, speed and grace of movement that should be natural.

The Alexander Technique is not widely practised in Ireland, but is a method suitable for all ages, with special applications for children.

List of Practitioners

The Society of Teachers of the Alexander Technique, (S.T.A.T.) is the practitioners' association in Ireland and Britain for qualified teachers of the Alexander Technique. Further information is available from: 10, London House, 266, Fulham Rd., London SW10 9EL. Tel. London 351 0828.

Cork:
Mrs. Jerilyn Scott, S.T.A.T., "Pigges Eye", South Schull, Co. Cork. Tel. 028-28429.
Dublin:
Mr. Frank Kennedy, S.T.A.T., 35, Callary Rd., Mount Merrion, Co. Dublin. Tel. 01-882446; Douglas T. Fraser, S.T.A.T., 32, Upr. Baggot St., Dublin 4. Tel. 01-683996.

Biofeedback

by Anne Gallagher

Biofeedback has been referred to as the teaching mirror. With the use of modern technology, stress levels are scientifically measured by placing sensors on the relevant areas and are shown on a monitor. Skin temperature, galvanic skin response and muscle tension are indicators of stress. With this information, an experienced therapist can teach you to control these levels putting you in control of your stress and your body.

Under the direction of the biofeedback expert who identifies your stress and teaches the relevant technique and by watching your body's responses, you learn control and ultimately need neither therapist or equipment. You have learned a technique for life.

There are over 50 conditions which can be successfully treated by biofeedback, e.g. anxiety, panic attacks, phobias, irritable bowel syndrome, high blood pressure, cardiac incidence and even the immune system resulting in fewer colds and infections. Biofeedback commenced in the U.S.A. in the 50's and with the development of technology has become more widely used and more efficient.

With the use of biofeedback instrumentation a build up of stress can be detected long before you have any symptoms, physical or emotional. This makes biofeedback a very useful technique in preventative medicine. Stress analysis or screening is at least as important as any other routine check up.

Biofeedback therapy is medically approved and is used in most leading clinics worldwide. It is a safe therapy and can replace or at least reduce medication.

Chapter Four

HOMOEOPATHY

I would like to thank Dr. Brian Kennedy, Dr. Elizabeth Ogden, and Lloyd Smith, whom I consulted for this article.

Samuel Hahnemann (1755-1843), the father of Homoeopathy, wrote in 1833:

> 'The old school physician . . . would not listen to any minute detail of all the circumstances of his case by the patient; indeed he frequently cut him short in his relation of his sufferings, in order that he might not be delayed in the rapid writing of his prescription . . . and still less did he make a note in writing of them. On seeing the patient again several days afterwards, he recollected nothing concerning the few details he had heard at the first visit (having in the meantime seen so many other patients labouring under different affections); . . . At subsequent visits he only asked a few general questions, went through the ceremony of feeling the pulse at the wrist, looked at the tongue, ...and, with a graceful bow, he hurried off to the fiftieth or sixtieth patient he had to visit, in this thoughtless way, in the course of that forenoon . . .'[1]

It seems that there is a great number of old school physicians practising in surgeries and hospitals to this day and since my own reaction to that mode of practice is less courteous than Dr. Hahnemann's, let us see instead what Homoeopathy offers!

Samuel Hahnemann was a physician and the initiator of homoeopathic medicine. He was also a linguist and a highly skilled pharmacist. His major philosophical work, *The Organon of Medicine* was completed thirty years before Pasteur established the *germ theory* of disease. (See p. 75) Medical practises in Hahnemann's time included *phlebotomy*; the cutting of veins to release unhealthy blood, leeches were

---

1   *The Organon of Medicine*, (6th Edition) by Samuel Hahnemann. Trans. William Boericke, M.D. (Boericke and Tafel, Philadelphia, 1952.)

also attached to the body to suck out the disease, and purgatives and emetics were used to expel the 'harmful forces'. Disease was often epidemic, notably cholera, and Hahnemann worked to find a better way.

The word *Homoeopathy* has its roots in the Greek words *Homois* which means similar to, and *Pathos*, suffering. Hahnemann termed the other prevalent medical method *Allopathy*, *Allo* meaning different from. In Homoeopathy, it is *The Vital Force* that regulates the healthy body and it is The Vital Force that responds to disease. The symptoms of an illness and the suffering of *The Life Force* are one and the same. Rather than suppressing symptoms, as in allopathic medicine, Homoeopathy works with The Vital Force, treating like with like. The *totality of symptoms* is gathered by physician and patient together and a remedy which induces the very same symptoms in the healthy body is given.

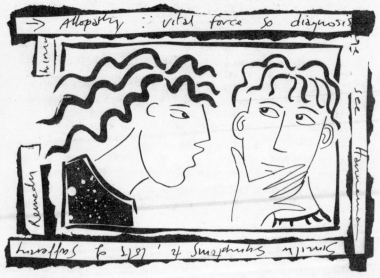

A bit of Philosophy

Hahnemann worked on the basis that it is not the body that becomes ill, physical symptoms are merely the signs that the force which animates and vitalises the human body is suffering. He developed remedies on the same principle — that medicinal substances have essential qualities which will neutralise illness, permitting *The Vital Force* to function correctly.

In homoeopathy, practitioners work, not with the visible, material content of medicines, but with their dynamic principles. The philosophy of this method was very much at odds with the thinking of Hahnemann's contemporaries and is still at odds with orthodox medical science. It works with the higher laws of nature, the laws governing the essence of things and is, in a way, closer to those branches of modern-day Physics that are primarily concerned with energy rather than with matter.

It is a measure of the effectiveness of Homoeopathy that it has survived through the era in history when the human race has been primarily concerned with gaining control over the visible material world. However, the ability to empirically observe is a function of the instrumentation used in observation and in contemporary science we learn more and more about less and less!

Dynamic Remedies

Dynamic remedies are derived from plant, mineral and animal sources and are tested and prepared with special methods such as *succussion* and *trituration*. Many remedies are derived from plants previously known and used in Herbal Medicine. Succussion (or shaking) is used for soluble substances. The medicinal substance in a material dose is diluted and succussed through a neutral alcohol base. This process is carried out until the imprint of the medicinal substance has been transferred into the solution. Trituration (pounding and grinding) is the method used to release the properties of non-soluble substances into a base of sugar of milk. By these and other methods, the remedy is potentised. The process is clearly not one of simple dilution and was developed empirically as a way of producing smoother and longer lasting results.

It is the understanding of Classical Homoeopathy that when a remedy or medicinal drug is used to suppress symptoms, the suffering may re-emerge in another form, and another, until it is addressed accurately. While Homoeopathic remedies are not toxic in the same way as medicinal drugs, The Vital Force will respond to them by generating new symptoms if they are incorrectly used. It is arguable that if Homoeopathic remedies are used over a long period of time to suppress symptoms i.e. to treat disease and not the patient — stress is created and side-effects can result.

The remedies used in Homoeopathy have been developed following clinical trials of the substances used. Hahnemann, his colleagues and successors, themselves took the substances and observed their effects on the healthy body. In their clinical trials they used, and in fact were the first to use, the 'double blind' method of observation. That is, that the reactions of two separate groups of participants to a stimulus are observed and both observers and participants are unaware which group is having the active stimulus. There are variations in this method, for example, one group may be given a placebo (i.e. a non-stimulant substance such as a sugar pill) and told that it is a strong substance while the other group may be told nothing. In this way the degree to which recipients' subjective expectations affect their reactions may also be assessed. This method of observation is now widely used in clinical medical and psychological studies and experiments.

One of the strongest counterclaims to the efficacy of dynamic remedies has been that they merely produce a *placebo* result, i.e. that they work because the person taking them believes that they will work, and that a sugar-pill or other non-medicinal substance would be equally efficacious. Two recently conducted experiments exploring the effectiveness of dynamic remedies are given below. These suggest that the remedies are biologically active and further research including sensitive immunological studies are now in progress.[2]

2   *The Difficulty with Homoeopathy.* A Paper presented at the British Pharmaceutical Conference Manchester, 14th September 1987, by David Taylor Reilly MRCP MRCGP MFHom RCCM/MRC Research Fellow and Morag A.Taylor, B. Sc.(Hons) RCCM/MRC Research Associate, University Department of Medicine, Glasgow Royal Infirmary, Glasgow.

Homoeopathic diagnosis

In order to effectively treat a patient, the Homoeopath must make a correct diagnosis, must have a knowledge of the medicines applicable and must select the remedy in the right dose. In Classical Homoeopathy, only one remedy is given, the Homoeopath aiming for the essential factor/s in the patient's conditions by using a remedy that is similar in its essence. Knowledge of the remedies is derived from clinical experience during training and from *The Materia Medicus*, a directory of remedies, giving detailed account of each remedy's effects. Computerised directories of symptoms and remedies may also be used.

The Totality of Symptoms

The phrase 'totality of symptoms' is used to describe the Classical Homoeopathic approach to diagnosis. In diagnosing, the Classical Homoeopath notes, in writing, each symptom described. Where there is a headache, the location of the pain and its nature — throbbing, piercing, blinding, etc. is noted. Where there is a temperature or cold, the patient's subjective experience is also noted. Loss of appetite; sleeplessness; lack of energy; the bowel motions; and so forth are noted with equal attention. Life-Style; environment; dietary habits; age; and sexual activity are also taken into account.

This picture of the symptoms of illness defines the disease, but also gives an understanding of how that person's constitution responds to disease. The patient's symptoms are seen not only as being caused in the first place by the disease, but also as indicators of the person's response. From the totality of symptoms, the Homoeopath goes on to ascertain how much of what has been said was peculiar to the person in his or her healthy state and what symptoms are the response of the vital force to disturbance of its functioning. Physical symptoms, the state of mind and way of being of the patient are all regarded as integral to the 'totality of symptoms', integral aspects of the person. Diagnosis and remedies given address themselves equally to these aspects.

Treating the patient, not the symptoms

In his early work, Hahnemann argued that, with the exception of the childhood illnesses, each instance of an illness needed to be understood and treated as an isolated, individual malady, for two reasons. First, because each occurrence takes its own particular form, and secondly because of the different constitution of each person. Later, Hahnemann identified patterns among diseases and types of human constitutions, while retaining the principle that there is no real cure for any disease without a strict particular treatment (individualisation) of each case of disease.

Either or/either and ...

Homoeopathy was developed before the microscope, the x-ray, the blood-pressure gauge, blood tests, the intravenous drip, antibiotics, psychotherapy, and the host of other diagnostic and therapeutic methods now available. Dynamic remedies are often used in conjunction with such techniques, and in the listings at the end of this section the different approaches of each practitioner listed are given. The degree of compatibility between Homoeopathy and other medical practises is a matter of debate that cannot be concluded here.

Homoeopathy has had great success in the treatment of disease, most notably in the cholera epidemic of 1831/32. By 1900 there was an estimated 15,000 practising Homoeopaths in the U.S.A., all of whom were MDs. They comprised approximately one sixth of the medical profession. Subsequently, The American Medical Association was formed with the clear objective of banning Homoeopaths from hospitals. By 1976, the number of Homoeopaths in the U.S.A. had fallen to 225 registered practitioners and there were no training schools.

This trend is gradually reversing itself. Following the establishment of the *germ theory* and the consequent burgeoning of the pharmaceutical industry, the idea that there was a specific drug to be found for specific diseases dominated medical research and practice. In response to disease in epidemic proportions, medicine developed on a mass basis. As we become aware of the dangers of drug-dependence, it seems that we turn again to methods of treatment that are more harmonious with our environment and with the body. Medical science has also recognised the success of treatments that accept the existence of The Vital Force, such as Homoeopathy and others outlined in this book. It remains to be seen how this recognition will develop — already in Scotland one tenth of G.P.s are trained in simple Homoeopathy with an appreciation of the complexities and potential of advanced homoeopathic prescribing.

First Aid Homoeopathy

Some dynamic remedies are freely available in wholefood shops and other outlets. Generally, it is remedies that have a wide application that are available in low doses in this way and there is a tradition of using the remedies for First Aid and for relief that dates from the frontier medicine of the U.S.A. Booklets are also available to help in the selection of such remedies. It is arguable, however, that the over-use of remedies on a mass basis is not Homoeopathy, that they are merely being used as a substitute for medical drugs such as Aspro which are also widely used to suppress 'minor' symptoms. Homoeopathic treatment of illness, properly speaking, involves correct diagnosis, knowledge of the remedies applicable and selection of the right dosage. While there is a range of Homoeopathic remedies that have wide applicability, it is common sense that they should not be used over and over again for recurring, or for varying, symptoms.

Case Studies

The following observations by Dr. Elizabeth Wright-Hubbard in the 1930s illustrate the Homoeopathic approach in the pre-antibiotic era. Dr. Wright-Hubbard first trained and worked as a medical or allopathic doctor in the U.S.A. She later studied Homoeopathy and is renowned for her work as a Homoeopath.

In a hospital ward there are three patients, all of whom have been admitted with pneumonia and who are receiving identical treatment. However, they are all suffering the illness in different ways:

The first patient is a strapping man who contracted pneumonia suddenly at midnight and was immediately admitted to Hospital. He is in mortal terror that he will die by noon the next day, and in fact he did die at that time. The Homoeopathic remedy in his case would be Aconite, indicated by the abrupt onset of the condition, fear of death and suitability for use in the early stages of a febrile illness.

The second patient is besotted, lying on his side, with his hand pressed against his chest. He lies motionless and gulps down two or three glasses of water at long intervals. He is sensitive to light and irritable on being approached. The Homoeopathic remedy would be Bryonia, indicated by pains aggravated by movement, copious thirst for water and irritability.

The third patient is very, very restless, especially in the evening and keeps calling for cold milk. His remedy would by Rhus-T, indicated by restlessness, relief of pain by movement and thirst for cold milk.

Vaccination

On the surface, there is a similarity between the theory behind vaccination and the theory behind Homoeopathy. A vaccination is the introduction into the system of mild forms of the bacteria or viruses prevalent in a disease so that the body will develop anti-bodies to the disease itself. Homoeopathy is the introduction of substances into the body showing symptoms of illness which cause like symptoms in a healthy person. That is as far as the comparison goes. There are many medics and parents who seriously question the value of vaccination as well as studies which call this practice into question and long running controversies have ensued.

One argument against vaccination, and one with which, as a parent, I concur, is that some childhood illnesses can help the child to mature, physically and emotionally. Often a healthy child becomes ill when he or she needs to enter a new stage in development and can be seen to acquire new and dramatic motor or social skills afterwards. The decision to vaccinate or not is by no means a simple one and it is worthwhile to discuss this with an experienced practitioner of parallel medicine as well as with an open-minded G.P. or Public Health Nurse. The option I have taken is to have vaccination against those illnesses whose consequences are extremely dangerous, or which I felt I could not nurse at home. The World Health Organisation maintains that 'the best vaccine against common infectious diseases is an adequate diet'.

References

Samuel Hahnemann, His Life and Works, by Richard Haehl, M.D., Vols 1 and 2. (Homoeopathic Publishing Company, London.)
'Vaccination — A Difficult Decision' leaflet produced by The Society of Homoeopaths, 2, Artizan Road, Northampton, NN14HU.
Everyday Homoeopathy, by David Gemmell (Beaconsfield)
Is Homoeopathy a Placebo Response? A Controlled Trial of Homoeopathic Potency, with Pollen in Hayfever as Model, by David Reilly MRCP, Morag Taylor, B.Sc., Charles McSharry, Ph.D. Tom Aitchison, B.Sc. (The Lancet No. 8512, Vol. 2 for 1986, London.)

Listing of Homoeopaths

The following list of Homoeopaths, and the descriptions, have been extracted by permission of the individual practitioners and the Homoeopathic Association of Ireland (HAI) from the HAI's annual booklet, *Homeopathy in Ireland*. The HAI is not a practitioners' organisation or a professional body, but exists to promote Homoeopathy. Membership is open to the public. Further information about the HAI is available from Jonathan Griffith, Blessington, Co. Wicklow. Tel. 045-65575.

Professional Homoeopaths
A Professional Homoeopath is someone who has completed a 3 for 4 year course, generally part-time, in Homoeopathy and basic medical science.

Patrick Brosnan, M.H.S. Reflexologist and Homoeopath, Tubridmore, Ardfert, Co. Kerry. Tel. 061-53890; Mary Dolan, Classical Homoeopath (L.C.H.), 26, Shelbourne Park, Limerick. Tel. 066-52169; Nuala Eising, Classical Homoeopath and Rebirther, Caherawoneen, Kinvara, Co. Galway. Tel. 091-37382; Lillian Van Eyeken, Classical Homoeopath (Holland), 69 Parc na gCaor, Moycullen, Co. Galway. Tel. 091-85367; Olive E. Kelly, D. Hom. Med., M.S.H.P.(London), S.R.N., Reflexologist, 32, Strand St., Clogherhead,

Drogheda, Co. Louth. Tel. 041-22702; William Kirkamm, Dip. Hom. Ph. D Hom. (London), Kiladoon, Westport, Co. Mayo. Tel. 098-68656.

Homoeopathic Doctors

A homoeopathic doctor is a fully qualified medical doctor who has specialised in Homoeopathy. The most readily available courses for doctors are those run by the Faculty of Homoeopathy in Glasgow.

Dr. Elizabeth Ogden, 29, Pembroke Park, Dublin 4. Tel. 01-680342; Dr. Goodwin McDonnell, 3, Upper Ely Place, Dublin 2. Tel. 01-616844; Dr. Brendan Fitzpatrick, 115 Morehampton Road, Dublin 4. Tel. 01-697768; Dr. Richard Fitzpatrick, 196, Upper Glenageary Road, Dublin. Tel. 01-854709; Dr. Martin Dekkers, Reenroe, Drimoleague, Co. Cork Tel.028-31364; also:5, Sydney Place, Cork, Tel. 021-506077; see also Acupuncture; Dr. Bas Van Eynatten, 5, Sydney Place, Wellington Road, Cork. Tel. 021-506077; Dr. Madeline Gordon, 119, Meadow Grove, Dundrum, Dublin 18. Tel. 01-986365; Dr. Brian Kennedy, 32, Upper Baggot Street, Dublin 4. Tel. 01-683996; Dr. James Dolan, 4c Olympia House, 61-63 Dame St., Dublin. Tel. 01-773591; Dr. Myles Frankel, Kilbrack, Doneraile, Co. Cork Tel. 022-24146; also: 1, Charleston Road, Rathmines, Dublin 6. Tel. 01-975666.

Natural Medicine Practitioners using Homoeopathy

Some Natural Medicine practitioners use methods from a variety of therapies other than their own. What is important is that the practitioners restrict themselves within the limits of their knowledge. It cannot be stressed enough that the unmonitored treatment of serious illness by unqualified practitioners is not advisable. In the following list of practitioners who use Homoeopathy in their practice, we (the HAI) have found it advisable to state the qualification of the practitioners and/or their experience, because standards of practice and training vary and one cannot necessarily be guaranteed the basic level of medical knowledge and expertise that is taken for granted with medical doctors.

Nigel Griffith, Primary Care Therapist, (7 years), Alta Vista, Sheestown, Kilkenny. Tel. 056-65402; Helen Grossman, Heilpraktierin (Germany), Clenor, Doneraile, Co. Cork. Tel. 022-24273; Brunhilde Keogh, Herbalism, Homoeopathy, Aromatherapy, Physiotherapy, "Annaville", Brittas, Co. Dublin. Tel.01-582351; Anthony Larkin, Reflexology. Chiropody, Homoeopathy, 41, Parkfield, New Ross. Tel. 051-22209; Christine Maxwell, Dip. Phytotherapy, Medical Herbalist (5 years), Dulcamara, Modeshill,

Mullinahone, Co. Tipperary. Tel. 052-53256; Ann Power, MBAHCh, MSRI,LCh, Homoeopathic Chiropodist, (5 years), 15, Kenilworth Road, Rathmines, Dublin. Tel. 01-974596; Ronald Turner, Acupuncture, Homoeopathy (V) (12 years), Cluain Ard, Stillorgan Road, Dublin. Tel. 01-884327.

Doctors using Homoeopathic medicines in their practice.

An increasing number of doctors are using Homoeopathic Medicines to a limited extent in their practices. Some sophisticated and controversial diagnostic equipment is becoming increasingly available. An example of this is Vega Testing, which is a diagnostic technique based on electric readings, which may indicate the use of a specially formulated remedy as part of the information provided. The letter 'V' after the practitioner's name indicates that Vega Testing is carried out.

Editor's note: Readers should note that Vega testing has recently become controversial in relation to both the expense and the accuracy of this method.

Dr. Paschal Carmody,(V), Thomas St., Killaloe, Co. Clare. Tel. 061-76349; Dr. John Clements, 70, Ranelagh Village, Dublin 6. Tel. 01-604810; see also acupuncture; Dr. M. Hayes, 104, Navan Road, Dublin 7. Tel. 01-387291; Dr. Lacey, (V), 185 Clonsilla Road, Blanchardstown, Dublin. Tel. 01-217365; Dr. M. Maguire, (V), 31, Hazelwood Court, Dublin 5. Tel. 01-471444; Dr. Colman Walsh, 12, Mart Street, Clonmel, Co. Tipperary. Tel. 052-21288; Dr. H.L.Webb, (V), "Knockoulart", Shankill, Dublin. Tel. 01-824602.

CENTRES

The Irish School of Classical Homoeopathy, which is based in Dublin, commenced classes on 25th January 1990.It provides a 4 year part-time training course in Classical Homoeopathy. Further information is available by writing to: The Irish School of Classical Homoeopathy, 29/30 Dame St., Dublin 2.

The Dublin Forum for Homoeopathic Medicine is a study group of doctors who are interested in Homoeopathic Medicine. The Membership has a wide range of expertise, from newcomers, to experienced practitioners. The forum aims to create a supportive environment for doctors who wish to use Homoeopathic medicines as a complementary therapy e.g. in general practise and also provides a venue for the continuing education of full time consultant Homoepathic physicians. Convenor: Dr. Brian Kennedy, 32, Upper Baggot St., Dublin 4. Tel. 01-683996.

The Burren College of Homoeopathy offers a four year part-time training in Classical Homoeopathy with a particular emphasis on the development of counselling skills. Courses will commence in October 1990. For further information contact: Nuala Eising, Caherawoneen, Kinvara, Co. Galway. Tel. 091-85367.

Northern Ireland Practitioners

Framar Natural Health Clinic, Dr. Frank Maconaghle, 595, Lisburn Rd., Belfast BT9 7GS. Tel. Belfast 681018/694210; Consultant Homoeopath and Herbalist. Reflexologist also available. Health assessment and counselling, Hair analysis, Massage, Allergy testing. Dr. John Murphy, 18, Killinchy St., Comber, Co. Down. Tel. Comber 872727; also Bio-energetics, Computer Testing, Allergy testing, Acupuncture, Manipulation, Shiatsu, Do-in, Radionics.

The Northern Ireland Homoeopathic Society (NIHS), is also an organisation which aims to disseminate knowledge of Homoeopathy among the public and at Government level. Membership is open to the public, contact The Secretary, NIHS, 32, Vauxhall Park, Belfast 9.

Doctors practising in Northern Ireland who are interested in Homoeopathy can contact: Dr. Annabelle Duff, Coagh, Co. Tyrone. Tel. Coagh 37467.

Chapter Five

DIET and NUTRITION

I would like to thank Anne Hyland, Carmel Kelleher, Cecilia Armelin, Coilin Uí hAiseadha and Bernadette Connolly-Martin for their help with this article.

Food in Context

Diet and Nutrition is one of the most debated aspects of health care and there is an awareness of the importance of a healthy balanced diet in every type of medical practice, alternative or mainstream. Yet, world hunger is a reality and one that is unacceptable, particularly when placed alongside the superpowers' defence budgets. Even in relatively wealthy countries health problems are caused or aggravated by lack of good quality food among the low-paid and unemployed and by over-eating among the wealthy. In every income-bracket, health problems arise from preservatives, colouring and sweetening agents when the health is already impaired, although the only symptoms may be tiredness or apathy. Even healthy foods such as fresh fruit and vegetables are not always free from artificial and toxic substances since these are introduced to the food-chain by industrial pollution or by the food industry itself in the form of artificial fertilisers, pesticides and weed-killers. For example in the United States, a large organic farm recently produced watermelons double the average size — not because of organic growing methods, but because of radiation from a nearby Uranium mine.

Although the Green Movement is growing and spreading awareness, it seems that this awareness is split — when we discuss war, separately from pollution or poverty. When we discuss food or diet, we generally do so in terms of the individual, or in terms of the family unit. When dietary therapy is used to treat people, an individually tailored diet is essential. But if diet is to be preventative of illness, the way in which food is grown, processed and distributed must be changed, as we will see in the next section. This is a social, political and economic process, as well as a matter of individual change and awareness.

When Irish supermarkets recently undercut rivals' prices for bread, many commentators expressed concern that price increases would follow and as a result poorer families would not be able to afford to buy bread. White bread is not high in nutritional value as it is highly processed and contains additives. The same is true of many other foodstuffs in the lower price range.

Perhaps one of the reasons that food is seen as a personal question is that many people express emotional and psychological disturbances through eating disorders. Food has deep emotional/psychological associations with the basic need to be nurtured. In infancy, we do not distinguish on any level between physical needs and emotional needs and this can carry over into adulthood. Food is then used to compensate for insufficient nurturing on the emotional level and this is often a factor for people who tend to overeat or who yearn for sweet foods. The tendency to undereat can be seen as a refusal or inability to nurture oneself and can be rooted in guilt feelings, or in anger towards or denial of the self. This is a complex area and when severe eating disorders

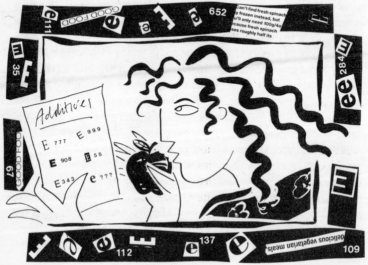

such as anorexia nervosa or bulimia occur it is advisable to seek the help of a suitably qualified counsellor or psychotherapist. (see Chap. 10)

In addition to the recognised problems associated with food, such as those mentioned above, one can also see tendencies, or patterns, that are not conducive to good health. How often do we reach for chocolate to compensate for a stressful situation, forget to eat or eat hurriedly while working on a project that will gain us approval or recognition? Self-help in these instances can begin with awareness and acceptance of our emotional needs and with consciously eating well, both for enjoyment as well as out of necessity.

Changing one's own or one's family's diet, for health reasons, environmental reasons, or both is not easy. It can be quite an experience to tour a supermarket with the objective of filling a family-sized trolley with food that is ideologically and nutritionally sound! With a list of unapproved or toxic E-numbers in one hand, list of required nutritional content for family members of different ages beneath it, one toddler in the shopping-trolley, another swinging from it — it seems so much easier to reach for the nearest food than to ask whether or not the apples have been sprayed with carcinogens (substances that can cause cancerous cells to form) to keep them shiny while on display.

For me, a change in diet was necessary as part of a programme of treatment for a skin condition called psoriasis. Dietary therapy can help alleviate the symptoms of many conditions, (e.g. asthma, arthritis, colitis, eczema, migraine, lethargy). Dietary improvements will certainly increase energy levels and general health. Dietary change, however, involves a lot of conscious effort, particularly in the early stages. A degree of dietary change will also accompany the advice and treatment of most practitioners of natural healing methods — rare is the person whose body has not suffered dietary excesses of one form or another, and even rarer, the person whose body can digest and eliminate poor food over a long period of time without some health problems occurring.

Where there is ill-health and dietary change is required, it is advisable to consult a qualified dietary therapist — to treat ill-health it may be necessary to eliminate a large number of foods from the diet and vitamin and mineral supplements may be needed for balanced intake.

All 'healthy' foods are not permissible on a treatment diet, in fact it is the appropriate use of healthy food with suitable management that enables detoxification and elimination thereby allowing the curative powers of the body to work. The whole process can be slow to complete, but the initial dietary change brings about dramatic results for most people. Dietary therapy is drug free but can and often does include the use of herbs, skin brushing and other adjuncts. Often, the body responds to extra help and this is where professional help which adheres to naturopathic principles will provide the smoothest course of action.

The requirements will vary from person to person, according to their health, age, weight, sex, etc. so it is advisable to consult a professional.

Some Don'ts

Although it can be alarming to discover the 'don'ts' in one's diet, it is important to look not just at one's own diet, but at the foods most commonly eaten by the population as a whole. A substantial amount of our national diet is made up of foods which have been over-refined or that contain additives, creating two types of problems:

Firstly, many foodstuffs are no longer 'whole', having had fibre, vitamin, and/or mineral content drastically reduced during processing. Secondly, food is added to; for taste, to make it last longer, look better, etc. The body cannot absorb and eliminate rich or additive-laden foods completely, and so its residues remain in the system. Such residues can be toxic or can accumulate in the blood circulatory system, in the lymphatic system, in the stomach and bowels, in the liver and kidneys, or in more than one of these organs and systems. A diet which is high in these types of foods leads initially to sluggish functioning of the body, and later to more serious health problems. The foods listed below feature prominently in the Irish diet. An excess of any one can be problematic and when these make up a major part of a diet, they are clearly unhealthy.

Dairy produce. Studies have shown that the dairy content of the European diet has soared in the last 5 generations and the high protein, vitamin and mineral content of dairy produce is widely known. However, many nutritionists believe that it plays too great a part in the average diet. One theory is that the body is not equipped to digest or eliminate the fats contained in dairy produce in the quantities commonly ingested nowadays. As a result, it is said, dairy produce can contribute to mucous conditions in childhood and to other conditions that do not emerge until adulthood when residues have accumulated, putting strain on the heart, digestive system, etc.

White sugar and white flour have both been refined to a degree that drastically reduces their vitamin and mineral content, providing inadequate material for the body's needs. White sugar, in order to be digested, drains the body of the B vitamins and magnesium creating a deficiency that affects the digestive system and also leads to mood swings, headaches and depression.

Cakes and sweets all contain at least one of the above as well as high levels of additives. Fancy foods contain the most E-numbers and preservatives. A list of E-numbers is given at the end of this chapter.

Meats, as well as dairy products, frequently contain high levels of antibiotic and hormonal residues from drugs given to livestock. While it is argued that they are present in amounts so small that they could not affect individual health, the cumulative effect over generations is virtually impossible to calculate.

Fruit and vegetables which have been artificially grown cannot compensate for the deficiencies of the bulk foods above. Artificial fertilisers increase the water content and thus the size of fruit and vegetables, but can actually reduce their vitamin and mineral content, while pesticides add toxins and kill off important health giving bacteria.

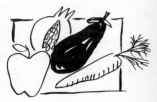

Tea and coffee are both addictive, creating a short-lived lift in energy levels followed by a sharp dip, so that our immediate reaction is to crave for another cup! They stimulate the body to use up its reserves of energy and are often used during a busy working day, at home, at the office, factory or wherever as a substitute for food. If taken when the body should be resting, the body's natural cleansing process is prevented from functioning. Over a period of time, the effects of tea and coffee include constant tiredness, moodiness, anxiety and tension, as well as an accumulation of waste matter in the body.

These are some foodstuffs which feature most often in the daily diet in Ireland. It seems that we are forced to face the reality that such a diet causes problems in individual health, in the health of future generations and that the methods used in their production are often pollutant. It is certainly time that we instigated change not just as individuals, but as a society.

Some elements of a healthy diet

Whole foods and organically grown fruit and vegetables are becoming more widely available. But it is nonetheless quite a shock to examine the household or individual diet and it is difficult to change to a wholefood diet since shopping, preparation and cooking all have to change too. These are some suggestions that can be quite easily and gradually introduced to most households. The suggestions given are intended as a guideline and not as a way of treating illness:

Use whole grains and cereals rather than potatoes, try out the different tastes and textures available. Whole grains and cereals include whole oats, pinhead oats, barley, long and short grain brown rice, millet, buckwheat. Wheat, as outlined above, is not easily digested and even real wheaten bread is

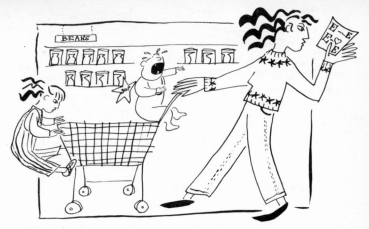

not a recommended staple food, although it is certainly an improvement on the white sliced pan.

Porridge made with whole oats or pinhead oats makes a hearty breakfast. If your children — or you — insist on a sweetener, try some mashed banana rather than sugar or honey.

Barley, a more indigenous grain than wheat, can be used in a variety of ways, (e.g. in soups, stews, or instead of rice or potatoes).

Eat plenty of fresh vegetables and fruit, organically grown if possible. Rather than presenting a child who is used to sweets with a rather daunting, whole and unpeeled apple or orange, give slices or segments, making sure that the fruit is ripe and tasty. Peel apples and pears for very young children, and when eating unpeeled fruit, always wash and wipe it well.

Cut down on salt, its essential components are already present in many foods. It is an unnecessary ingredient and one that creates health problems when used excessively. Sea salt, or condiments containing it, such as natural soysauce or miso, can be taken in moderation instead. Many tinned and processed foods contain a lot of salt.

Minimise foods that are artificially refined or processed and that contain artificial additives. Beware of E-numbers — see list below. Natural substances such as monosodium glutomate can also be be used as preservatives, but are unhealthy in large amounts. Cut down drastically on foods that are high in saturated fats including meats, chocolate, confectionery, fries, dairy foods, chips, etc. and use good quality unrefined oils for cooking. Eat regularly, leaving time for digestion between meals. If you like or need to eat more often, snack on fruit, whole grains and cereals, nuts, seeds and dried fruit; take low-fat protein foods such as cottage cheese, natural live yoghurt, fresh fish, nuts and seeds; drink herbal teas or grain coffee instead of the usual.

Try the many kinds of beans that are available. The tinned variety can be sugar-free, but raw uncooked beans and pulses cost far less than tinned foods or meats. In a vegetarian, or semi-vegetarian diet, they are the main source of protein, but must be taken with grains to make up a source of complete protein (complete protein, i.e. protein equivalent to meat or fish in that it contains the full range of amino acids). Most beans need to be soaked overnight before cooking, butter beans are the exception. They make delicious stews, with vegetables and seasoned with herbs or spices.

Investigate the local wholefood shop — the atmosphere and staff are usually much more pleasant than the supermarket and a wide range of recipe books and leaflets are available. Introduce changes gradually, and don't guilt trip yourself — the habits of a lifetime are not suddenly swept away. After eating whole foods for a period of time the taste buds sharpen and can be trusted to tell what is needed. Cravings, on the other hand, tell what is being eliminated from the body, merely indicating what has already been taken to excess.

Macrobiotics

Macrobiotics is the basis of a healthy diet as outlined above, and plays a major part in the work of practitioners listed below. Macrobiotics is also a philosophical approach to food and to life that teaches harmony between the person and the environment. It is a tenet of macrobiotics that food gives more than vitamins, minerals and protein. Food is energy, and as an oriental philosophy, macrobiotics classifies food into *Yin* and *Yang*. Yin-Yang are the opposites inherent in life, Yin is heaven's force, Yang is earth's force. Yin foods make us spacey, nervous and anxious when taken in excess, Yang foods earth us, and make us aggressive. The following is a guide to the Yin-Yang of food. To think of one's food in terms of providing a balance of energy, as well as a balanced intake of various chemicals introduces a new perspective to diet, and one that is invaluable. Think about it the next time you contemplate a plate of chips with tomato sauce.

Very Yang: Refined salt, eggs, hard salty cheeses, red meat/fish, some drugs.

Mildly Yang: Unrefined salt, white meat/fish, shellfish, miso, shoyu, tamari.

More balanced: Whole cereal grains, beans, temperate climate vegetables, seeds, sea vegetables.

Mildly Yin: Temperate climate fruits, nuts, vegetable oils, non-stimulant drinks.

Very Yin: Sugar, honey, spices, milk, yogurt, cream, wines, spirits, stimulant drinks, most food additives, many drugs.

The Spirit of Cooking

by Anne Hyland

The following article has been reproduced form the Irish Holistic Health Association Newsletter. I am including it here with Anne's permission because it conveys the sense of good energy implicit in this approach to healthy eating.

There are many diets and special foods for improving our health. However, the most important ingredient is our way of cooking. Paying special attention to the origin and quality of our food offers us the best opportunity to adapt to changing circumstances in our environment and in our life. When we meet change, often our first reaction is to resist, and to indulge our desires as a way to escape what is actually happening.

By simplifying our eating habits, choosing basic cereals, fresh vegetables, and other natural foods, we can focus our energy effectively to overcome difficulties from change and sickness. The attention we give to choosing our food, with preparation, cutting and ways of cooking, creates an energy which changes our condition. When we ignore this attention, taking foods indiscriminately, our energy is lost and our condition weakens.

Creating a peaceful and happy environment in our kitchen is essential to good cooking. When we use the best fuel (solid fuel or gas), the best pots (heavy cast iron, enamel, or light stainless steel), good knives for cutting, we are already starting with the right effort. When we choose food of quality and know where it is coming from, how it is produced, we have the best ingredients. Now our mind is prepared for making a delicious meal.

Next we choose a variety of colours and flavours to combine. We plan a menu to suit our time and circumstances, to include some grain (barley, brown rice, millet or others), some green vegetables, some root vegetables. For flavour we add quality condiments like sea salt, natural soysauce or miso soy paste, in small quantity. A small amount of beans or lentils, seeds (sesame or sunflower) or nuts will complement the grain and vegetable dishes when we minimise the use of animal food and fish. All these need appropriate cooking and good chewing to absorb the best energy. Dried fruit and local and seasonal fruits provide sweetness. Sea vegetables provide minerals. Wholewheat pasta and occasional wholewheat breads provide variety to our base of whole cereal grains.

Whole cereal grains provide our stable base, our centre from which we can create endless variety with other legumes and vegetables. These foods develop the essential connection with the wisdom of our ancestors in adapting to our environment with a sense of freedom and gratitude for life.

List of E-numbers

(prepared by the Wales Ecology Party).

This list of food colourings and additives has been published by the Hospital Centre, Chaumont, France, based upon information from the Research Centre Hospital of Ville, France, to highlight the effects of colours and additives used in the food industry.

E100 Harmless
E101 Harmless
E102 Dangerous
(tartarine)
E103 Forbidden
E104 Suspect
E105 Forbidden
E110 Dangerous
(yellow)
E111 Forbidden
E120 Dangerous
E121 Forbidden
E122 Suspect
E123 Very Dangerous
E124 Dangerous (fizzy)
E125 Forbidden
E126 Forbidden
E127 Dangerous
E130 Forbidden
E131 Carcinogenic
E132 Harmless
E140 Harmless
E141 Suspect
E142 Carcinogenic
E150 Suspect
E151 Suspect
E152 Forbidden
E153 Suspect
E160 Harmless
E161 Harmless
E163 Harmless
E170 Harmless
E171 Suspect
E173 Suspect
E174 Harmless
E175 Harmless
E180 Suspect
E181 Forbidden
E200 Harmless
E201 Harmless
E202 Harmless
E203 Harmless
E210 Carcinogenic
E211 Carcinogenic
E212 Carcinogenic
E213 Carcinogenic
E214 Carcinogenic
E215 Carcinogenic
E217 Carcinogenic
E220 Destroys Vitamin
B12

E221 Intestinal
Disorder
E222 Intestinal
Disorder
E223 Intestinal
Disorder
E224 Intestinal
Disorder
E226 Intestinal
Disorder
E230 Skin Disorder
E231 Skin Disorder
E233 Skin Disorder
E236 Harmless
E237 Harmless
E238 Harmless
E239 Carcinogenic
E240 Suspect
E241 Suspect
E250 Blood Pressure
problems
E251 Blood Pressure
problems
E252 Blood Pressure
problems
E260 Harmless
E261 Harmless
E262 Harmless
E263 Harmless
E270 Harmless
E280 Harmless
E281 Harmless
E282 Harmless
E300 Harmless
E301 Harmless
E302 Harmless
E303 Harmless
E304 Harmless
E305 Harmless
E306 Harmless
E307 Harmless
E308 Harmless
E309 Harmless
E311 Skin Rash
E312 Skin Rash
E320 Cholesterol
E321 Cholesterol
E322 Harmless
E325 Harmless
E326 Harmless
E327 Harmless

E330 Carcinogenic
E330 Cold Sores
E331 Harmless
E332 Harmless
E333 Harmless
E334 Harmless
E335 Harmless
E336 Harmless
E337 Harmless
E338 Digestive
Disorder
E339 Digestive
Disorder
E340 Digestive
Disorder
E341 Digestive
Disorder
E400 Harmless
E401 Harmless
E402 Harmless
E403 Harmless
E404 Harmless
E406 Harmless
E407 Digestive
Disorder
E408 Harmless
E410 Harmless
E411 Harmless
E413 Harmless
E414 Harmless
E440 Harmless
E421 Harmless
E422 Harmless
E450 Digestive
Disorder
E461 Digestive
Disorder
E462 Digestive
Disorder
E463 Digestive
Disorder
E465 Digestive
Disorder
E466 Digestive
Disorder
E471 Harmless
E472 Harmless
E473 Harmless
E474 Harmless
E475 Harmless
E477 Suspect

Carcinogenic: Substance which can cause cancerous cells to form

Forbidden: Banned by the French Health Minister from 1 Jan 1977

Suspect: Suspect product with side effects currently under investigation

Destroys Vitamin B12: Vital to proper functioning of the nervous system.

Blood Pressure Problems: This substance is present in pre-cooked meats.

All these food additives are presently permitted in Britain and Ireland and are shown on food packs. Carefully choose the products you buy, avoiding foodstuffs containing any of the harmful or dubious additives or colourings referred to in the above list. Your health and that of your family depends on what kind of food you buy.

Practitioners

Medical Dietary Therapy

Cecilia Armelin, Senior Dietitian, B.Sc. Tel. 01-752355 (W)/01-682061 (H) for appointment; Dietary Counselling for adults, children and infants. Special interest in food intolerance and the medicinal qualities of foods. Nutritional advice to customers in The Hopsack, Rathmines, on alternate Saturdays. Green Party Spokeswoman on Food.

Bernadette Connolly-Martin, D. Th. D., "Slainte", Eaton Wood, Corbawn Lane, Shankill, Co. Dublin. Tel. 01-822132; Dietary Therapy — nutritional medicine following naturopathic principles and using adjuncts when necessary.

Veronica Crombie, 71, Pembroke Rd., Ballsbridge, Dublin 4. Tel. 01-602137; Nutritional Counsellor, Vegetarian and Wholefood Cookery teacher. Holds a

Diploma from the Kushi Institute in Boston.

Patricia Quinn, "Sunnyhill", Bohernabreena, Dublin 24. Tel. 01-513619; Nutritional Counsellor, S.R.N. and Midwife. Nutritional advice to customers in Nature's Way, ILAC Centre, Dublin — Wednesdays. Candida, Pre-menstrual tension, Menopause, Hyperactivity and Food Sensitivity in children.

General Dietary Advice and Cookery Teachers

Pauline Fitzmaurice, Ceres Wholefoods, Powerscourt Townhouse Centre, Dublin 2. Tel. 01-794292; general dietary advice in Ceres Wholefoods and holds Cookery Classes regularly. Telephone or drop in for further information.

Marliese Maguire, Tel. 01-484270; general dietary advice with a special emphasis on mothers and children. She cooks 'Open House' meals by arrangement, telephone to book.

Dorothee Dupont, Tel. 021-342794/066-58189; runs ten week introductory classes in Cork city, consisting of demonstrating food preparation with soups, grains, beans, sea-weeds, sugar-free desserts.

Teach Ban, 6, Parnell Rd., Harolds Cross, Dublin 6. Tel. 01-543943; Ann Currie and Patrick Duggan give Macrobiotic Consultations, Wholefood cookery classes are also held at Teach Ban.

Tony Quinn Health Stores and Nutritional Therapy; A full nutritional consultation at one of the Tony Quinn Centres costs £25 or £35 to include follow-up.

Holders of the Diploma in Holistic Dietetics (DHD)

The Diploma in Holistic Dietetics is issued by the Irish Health Cultural Association and is based on the Tony Quinn methods.

Cork:
Eileen Allen-Clair MIHCA, 54 Silverdale Ave., Ballinlough, Cork; Denis O'Callaghan MIHCA, 51 Clover Lawn, Skehard, Cork. Tel. 021-357947; Stacey Quinlivan MIHCA, 2 Avondale, Western Road, Cork; Tim Humphreys MIHCA, 20 Monard House, Whitechurch, Co. Cork. Tel. 021-503775; Mary O'Regan MIHCA, Ballinahina, Whitescross, Co. Cork. Tel. 021-88437.

Kerry:
Pam Pennings MIHCA, Upper Mount Coal, Listowel, Co. Kerry. Tel. 068-40168; David Sankar MIHCA, 5 Urban Tce., Boherbee, Tralee, Co. Kerry. Tel. 066-24035.

Kildare:
Ann Skelly MIHCA, 88 Glendale Est., Leixlip, Co. Kildare. Tel. 242308.

Kilkenny:
Mairead Burke MIHCA, Poulecapple, Callan, Co. Kilkenny. Tel. 052-53281h, 23211w.

Louth:
Mary McCumiskey MIHCA, Ballynamoney, Greenore, Dundalk, Co. Louth. Tel. 042-73257h, 041-37653w; David O'Connor MIHCA, Tony Quinn Centre, Jocelyn St., Dundalk, Co. Louth.

Monaghan:

Yvonne Thornton MIHCA, Yoga Therapist, Tony Quinn Centre, Carrickmacross, Co. Monaghan. Tel. 042-612884; Bernard Murphy MIHCA, Kilmactrasna, Carrickmacross, Co. Monaghan. Tel. 042-67172w.

Waterford:

Caroline Moran MIHCA, 5 Barronstrand St., Waterford. Tel. 051-76279.

Wicklow:

Marie Warren MIHCA, 49 Heather Vue, Greystones, Co. Wicklow. Tel. 877763.

Dublin County-South:

Liam McDonald MIHCA, Tony Quinn Centre, Dun Laoghaire; Jonathan Freestone MIHCA, 12 Grange Tce., Deansgrange Rd., Blackrock, Co. Dublin. Tel. 892694, 893955w; Mary O'Shea MIHCA, 2 Glenamena Grove, Blackrock, Co. Dublin. Tel. 691844; John Clarke MIHCA, 15 Clarinda Pk. West, Dun Laoghaire, Co. Dublin. Tel. 841860; Carole MacMahon MIHCA, 66 Marsham Ct., Stillorgan, Co. Dublin. Tel. 885833.

Dublin 4, 6 & 8:

Vivienne Tobin MIHCA, 92 Willfield Road, Dublin 4. Tel. 838550; Eileen Ryan MIHCA, 5 Richelieu Pk., Ballsbridge, Dublin 4. Tel. 691084; Edmund Wall MIHCA, 22 Shelbourne Road, Ballsbridge, Dublin 4. Tel. 603876; Patricia Wheeler MIHCA, 28 Kenilworth Road, Rathmines, Dublin 6. Tel. 960236; Patricia McKenna MIHCA, 2 Bloomfield Ave., Sth Circular Rd., Dublin 8. Tel. 543319.

Dublin 12, 14, 16 & 20:

Gerry Wilson MIHCA, Rathbeale Rd., Swords, Co. Dublin. Tel. 402852; Irene Jordan MIHCA, 51 Galtymore Close, Drimnagh, Dublin 12. Tel. 557440; Kay Farrell MIHCA, 21 Park Crescent, Kimmage, Dublin 12. Tel. 552895; Marie Brennan MIHCA, 18 Tonduff Close, Green Park, Walkinstown, Dublin 12. Tel. 513159; Laureanne Kelly MIHCA, 41 Whitebeam Rd., Clonskeagh, Dublin 14. Tel. 506594; Cyril Mahon MIHCA, 99 Glenvara Park, Ballycullen Road, Templeogue, Dublin 16. Tel. 942437; Marie McHugo MIHCA, 42 Manor Road, Palmerstown, Dublin 20. Tel. 264574.

Dublin County — North:

Michael Cantwell MIHCA, Haddon Lodge, Thormanby Rd., Howth, Co. Dublin. Tel. 322096; Siobhan Clifford MIHCA, 5 Church St., Howth, Co. Dublin. Tel. 323067; Dan J. Lucey MIHCA, 60 Biscayne, Malahide, Co. Dublin. Tel. 452005; Anne O'Donnell MIHCA, 26 Seabury Heights, Malahide, Co. Dublin. Tel. 450615; Bernadette Ui Obain MIHCA, 29 Forest Boulevard, River Valley, Swords, Co. Dublin. Tel. 405540.

Dublin 3, 5:

David Harding MIHCA, 25 Haddon Road, Clontarf, Dublin 3. Tel. 339544; Patricia Mulligan MIHCA, 44 Malahide Road, Clontarf, Dublin 3. Tel. 331485; Katherine Cooke MIHCA, 5 The Crescent, Fairview, Dublin 3. Tel. 337252; Geraldine Leggett MIHCA, 27 Woodbine Drive, Raheny, Dublin 5. Tel. 783484.

Dublin 7 & 9:

Vincent Harford MIHCA, Tony Quinn Centre, 66 Eccles St., Dublin 7; Maeve Macken MIHCA, 11 Sion Hill Road, Dublin 9. Tel. 378310; Mary Dolan MIHCA, 10 Park Drive Grove, Castleknock, Dublin 15. Tel. 204029; Mary O'Dea MIHCA, 55 Castleknock Elms, Castleknock, Dublin 15. Tel. 202144; Margaret Watts MIHCA, 15 Roselawn View, Castleknock, Dublin 15. Tel. 212573.

Overseas:
Andrew Moore MIHCA, 9 Namhaugh Island, Shepperton, Middlesex. Tel. 030932-244603.
Joan Langley MIHCA, De Lairessestraat 9, Eindhoven, The Netherlands.

SEAMUS CARTER
MASSAGE & BODYWORK TABLES LTD.

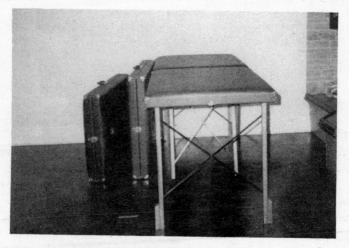

- Massage Tables
- Professional
- Portable
- Made to Individual Requirements
- Comfortable
- Beautiful
- Guaranteed

15 Woodlands Road, Johnstown Estate, Dunlaoghaire, Dublin.

Phone (01) 850087

Chapter Six

MASSAGE

by Judith Ashton

Judith Ashton practises and teaches massage in Dublin, working with individuals and groups. She also practises contact healing, psychotherapy and counselling, is a member of the National Federation of Spiritual Healers in England and has taught and worked in England, Greece and Scandinavia.

Of all the healing arts known to man, massage must be the oldest and most instinctive. What is more natural than to rub or stroke an area of the body that feels tense or aching? In today's stress filled world we all need to learn how to relax. The power of touch cannot be underestimated, a gentle loving touch or massage can dissolve both physical and psychological tensions and heal at the deepest levels.

Massage was an integral part of medical practise in many of the ancient cultures and civilisations of the world — it was used by Egyptians, Persians, Romans, Greeks, Japanese, Chinese, American Indians and Eskimos to name but a few. It was widely practised in Europe until the Middle Ages and the Reformation — this period represented a serious setback in the open practise and development of massage because of the repressive religious thinking of the time.

The Renaissance revived the interest in medicine and massage was once more acknowledged — we know that many of the European courts of this period had physicians who successfully incorporated massage into their treatments. Sadly, as time went on approaches to medicine have become less and less personal and more and more technical, mechanistic and drug oriented. It wasn't until the late 1800s that Peter Ling went to the Far East where he observed the daily practises and techniques of massage and it was from this that Swedish massage was developed as a physical treatment widely used in hospitals.

Today, with the great public demand for alternative therapies and preventative medicine, the benefits of massage are being widely recognised. On a purely physical level massage affects all the major systems in the body which includes the muscles, skin, lymph system, circulation etc. and can encourage the organs and systems to function effectively.

Massage is known to have a positive effect on high blood pressure, digestive disorders, muscular aches and pains, back problems, certain injuries, arthritis and rheumatism. It aids sleep, can help pain relief and general stress and tension to name but a few.

Most forms of massage aim to relax the body and in doing so can also relax the mind. When both mind and body are deeply relaxed the self-healing capacity of the physical body is encouraged, especially if the intention of the therapist is to unblock and channel energy. This is the aim of many types of massage, but the wider implications of touch cannot be under-estimated. A lot has been written about the physical response to touch, very little on the psychological significance of touch.

Touch is basic, simple, and universal. It cuts through race, colour and creed. It is direct communication and sadly we're mostly out of touch. Look at the language, especially English 'in touch', 'out of touch','it touches me','a touching moment', etc. Touch is a forgotten healing art, we've forgotten how to touch, where to touch and when to touch each other and we need to relearn it. The therapeutic use of hands is a universal human act, something we've forgotten in our admiration of mechanical technology. Touch is the most personally experienced of all the senses, after all it is the earliest sense to develop in the human embryo and the awareness of self is largely a matter of tactile experience.

Touch is not just a physical sensation it is always, and has to be regarded as, an emotional experience. It can't be always taken for granted that everyone has a positive attitude towards touch, hopefully most of us have had positive parenting and comforting, non-threatening physical contact with family and friends and thus regard touch as a source of pleasure. There has been an upsurge of interest and research into child abuse and statistics prove that many people have undergone painful, distressing and negative experiences to do with touch and physical abuse. For these people touch can be an extremely threatening way of being related to another person and this brings us to an awareness of physical and psychological boundaries and permission in relationship to touch.

Each of us has our own particular boundaries in relation to touch. We are very clear about who we allow to touch us, where they can touch us and how they can touch us. This comes back to the idea of permission and there are social rules and roles which abide in terms of touch. Touch will only be a positive, comforting way of relating if the person being touched feels positive and in control of the situation. Touch for many people is threatening because of its sexual connotations. They know only sexual touch.

The word massage in the West has for a long time been used within a sexual context — in fact serious massage has nothing to do with sex at all but more to do with healing and it is within this healing context that many practitioners are now working. Healing not only the body — if they are skilled, with an understanding of the mind-body connection, they can help heal inner emotional tensions by facilitating insights into the nature and origins of stress factors. Massage and touch can be a deeply moving even spiritual experience.

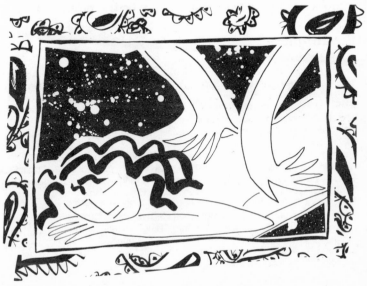

When you are being massaged you can feel extremely vulnerable and so it is important that you choose your practitioner carefully. Ensure that you feel confident and trusting with the person that you choose to work with and find out before your first meeting about their approach to their craft.

There are a variety of forms of massage. Reflexology, Shiatsu and Aromatherapy have been described separately. Some other forms are :

Swedish Massage: A set pattern of strokes designed to improve circulation and muscle tone.

Ki Massage Therapy: A combination of traditional massage techniques with healing, designed to put the person in contact with their energy (Ki) as developed by Tony Quinn.

Deep tissue massage/Rolfing: Designed to relax muscles and improve posture.

Remedial Massage: To improve mobility of muscles and joints usually in conjunction with exercises.

Biodynamic massage (Gerda Boyeson method): To dissolve inner tension of the whole body by following energy responses of the 'psycho-peristalsis'.

Touch for Healing (Judith Ashton): To create through the medium of touch, massage and communication an awareness of blockage and harmony of the mind/body/spirit.

Practitioners

Dublin:

Judith Ashton, 28, Seapoint Ave., Monkstown, Co. Dublin. Tel. 01-809630; Massage, bio-dynamic massage, Reichian bodywork, psychotherapy, counselling, stress-management, dream interpretation, energy work and contact healing; Pamela Butler,14, Belgrave Rd., Dublin 6. Tel. 01-977142; Therapeutic Massage; Philomena Brady, Natural Living Centre, 5, St. James Tce., Malahide, Co. Dublin. Tel. 01-452050. Holistic Massage, Aromatherapy, Yoga; Sarah Codd, 14, Woodlawn Park, Mounttown, Dun Laoghaire, Dublin. Tel. 01-843856; Healing Massage Therapy. Also at the Natural Living Centre, 5, St. James Tce., Malahide, Co. Dublin. Tel. 01-452050. Joan Davis, The Studio, rear 330 Harold's Cross Road. Tel. 908118; Shiatsu massage with a unique method of voice work (also Movement and Dance, see below); Roisin Hilliard, Natural Living Centre, 5, St. James Tce., Malahide, Co. Dublin. Tel. 01-452050; Holistic Massage; Tom Quinn, 15, Kincora Grove, Clontarf, Dublin 3. Tel. 332453; Therapeutic Massage, (relaxing), Holistic Massage, (relaxing). ITEC Massage, (vigorous); Mary Timmons, 22, Springhill Ave., Blackrock, Co. Dublin. Tel. 01-896555; Holistic Massage Therapy; Eileen Wetherall, 37, Dunville Avenue, Ranelagh, Dublin 6. Tel. 01-839330; Clinical Massage, also S.R.N.

Kildare:
Martina Moylan and Sr. Eileen Ryan, Convent of Mercy, Athy, Co. Kildare. Tel. 0507-31361; also Reflexology.

The Natural Therapy Centre provides courses in Aromatherapy and Massage. Massage Therapists who have trained there are listed below. Further information is available from : The Natural Therapy Centre, 12, Tivoli Tce. South, Dun Laoghaire, Co. Dublin. Tel. 01-809505.

Carlow:
Mary Attridge, Bagenalstown, Co. Carlow. Tel. 0503-57692.
Clare:
Vivienne Purcell, Ennis, Co. Clare. Tel. 065-21684.
Cork:
Catherine T.Rea, Mitchelstown, Co. Cork.
Dublin:
Mary Attridge, Raheny, Dublin. Tel. 0503-57692; Gerard Brennan, Rathcoole, Co. Dublin. Tel. 01-580524; Mary de Brun, Foxrock, Dublin 18. Tel. 01-883111; Anne Brophy, Castleknock, Dublin 15. Tel. 01-203720; Phyllis Byrne, 38, Seafield Road, Clontarf, Dublin 3; Ann Cahill, Merrion, Dublin 4. Tel. 01-698302; Gay Campion, Castleknock, Dublin 15. Tel. 01-214008; Eleanor Carpenter, Ranelagh, Dublin 6. Tel. 01-979691; Mary Cavanagh, Natural Therapy Centre, Dun Laoghaire, Co. Dublin. Tel. 01-809505; Suzanne Costello, Artane, Dublin 5. Tel. 01-474581; Kim Donohoe, Natural Therapy Centre, Dun Laoghaire, Co. Dublin. Tel. 01-809505; Deirdre Dooley, Rathfarnham, Dublin 14. Tel. 01-933806; Dolores Fahy, Ballsbridge, Dublin 4. Tel. 01-600311 Ext.3500; Marian Farrell, Blackrock, Co. Dublin. Tel. 01-831665; Adrienne Finnerty, Monkstown, Co. Dublin. Tel. 01-843634; Greg Gallagher, Dun Laoghaire, Co. Dublin. Tel. 01-855866; Dympna Hall, Rathfarnham, Dublin 16. Tel. 01-945601; Mary Hartnett, Stillorgan, Co. Dublin. Tel. 01-880193; Ann Healy, Rathfarnham, Dublin 16. Tel. 01-931732; Michelle Hetherington, Stillorgan, Co. Dublin. Tel. 01-889771; Paula Keegan, Sutton, Dublin 13. Tel. 01-326010; Margaret Kyne-Doyle, Loughlinstown, Co. Dublin. Tel. 01-823753; Kim Levingston, Dundrum, Dublin 14. Tel. 01-985573; Mary Lewellyn, Dublin 9. Tel. 01-315814; Suzanne Martin, Glenageary, Co. Dublin. Tel. 01-806762; Julie Meagher, Artane, Dublin 5. Tel. 01-310599; Fiona Merry, Blackrock, Co. Dublin. Tel. 01-882419; Rosemary McCarthy, Donnybrook, Dublin 4. Tel. 01-975808; Agnes McGuinness, Garristown, Co. Dublin. Tel. 01-354266; Patricia Moore, Killiney, Co. Dublin. Tel. 01-853076; Stan Moore, Loughlinstown, Shankill, Co. Dublin. Tel. 01-822948; Pauline Moriarty, Upper Kilmacud Road, Co. Dublin. Tel. 01-884348; Maria Murnane, Raheny, Dublin 5. Tel. 01-410536; Anne Murray, Churchtown, Dublin. Tel. 01-985600; Sean O'Riain, Monkstown, Co. Dublin. Tel. 01-843169; Mary O'Shea, Ranelagh, Dublin 6. Tel. 01-963137; Eithne Perry, Dundrum, Dublin 16. Tel. 01-951754; Francis Pierce, Sutton, Dublin 13. Tel. 01-326010; Ann Power, Drumcondra, Dublin. Tel. 01-375097; Imelda Prior, Merrion Road, Dublin 4. Tel. 01-838981; Brid Roe, Swords, Co. Dublin. Tel. 01-401181; Elizabeth Ruttledge, Cabinteely, Dublin 18. Tel. 01-856793; Ann O'Shanahan, Dundrum, Dublin 16. Tel. 01-953630; Seamas Sullivan, Dun Laoghaire, Co. Dublin. Tel. 01-805695; Mona Sweetman, Skerries, Co. Dublin. Tel. 01-491757; Sarah Treasy, Churchtown, Dublin 14. Tel. 01-980101; Sr. Brega

Whelan, Beaumont, Dublin 9. Tel. 01-379186; Christine Walsh, Rathfarnham, Dublin 16. Tel. 01-933215.

Kildare:
Kay Murphy, Naas, Co. Kildare. Tel. 045-66531.

Laois:
Bridie Grace, Portlaoise, Co. Laois. Tel. 0502-27092.

Longford:
Deirdre Leavy, Edgeworthstown, Co. Longford. Tel. 043-71156.

Louth:
Jacqueline Gough, Dunleer, Co. Louth. Tel. 042-72724; Dympna McGrath, Drogheda, Co. Louth. Tel. 041-31510; Roisin McGroder, Dunleer, Co. Louth.

Mayo:
Noeleen Cashin-Cafolla, Castlebar, Co. Mayo. Tel. 094-21542.

Offaly:
Sheila Keeneghan, Banagher, Co. Offaly. Tel. 0902-51383.

Tipperary:
Tina Hickey, Nenagh, Co. Tipperary. Tel. 067-32444; Maria O' Brien, Fetherd, Co. Tipperary. Tel. 052-31508.

Waterford:
Catherine Bell, Cork Road, Waterford. Tel. 051-75966.

Wicklow:
Angela M. Mahon, Bray, Co. Wicklow. Tel. 01-861687; Mary Shanley, Delgany, Co. Wicklow. Tel. 01-877722.

The Institute of Physical Therapy and Applied Science provides courses. Further information is available from The Institute, Sir Patrick Dun's Hospital, Grand Canal St., Dublin 2. Tel. 611666. Its founder, Anne Mangan is a medical massage therapist; 5 Bayview Lawns, Killiney. Tel. 01-821153; and at the Well Woman Centre, Leeson St., Dublin 2. Tel. 01-610083.

Northern Ireland Practitioners

Mary Grant, 111, Cliftonville Rd., Belfast BT14 6JQ. Tel. Belfast 753658; also practises and teaches Aromatherapy, is a Counsellor and the Co-ordinator of Lifespring. (see p. 207); Swami Gyanjyoti, 21, Hampton Park, Belfast BT7 3JN. Tel. Belfast 641052/693238; Also Metamorphic Technique; Brian McCrystal, The Natural Therapy Clinic, Pentagon House, Ballymena, Co. Antrim. Tel. Ballymena 49701; Also Aromatherapy, Reflexology, Physiotherapy, Health foods, essential oils, Bach flower remedies, natural medicines, etc. Will do home visits; Julie Murphy, 18, Killinchey St., Comber, Co. Down. Tel. Comber 872727; Also Naprapaony (gentle Spinal manipulation), Acupressure, Reflexology, Homoeopathy, applied Kinesiology; Sighla Mary O'Donoghue, Shambhala, 7, Ashley Gardens, Belfast BT15 4DU. Tel. Belfast 771104; Also Integration Counselling and Therapy; Evan Pamely, 108, Comber Rd., Killyleagh, Downpatrick BT30 9PG. Tel. Downpatrick 828307; Mary Peters Health Club, 37, Railway St., Lisburn, Co. Antrim. Tel. Lisburn 76411; Also specially designed exercise programmes, sauna and hydrotherapy pool.

Movement and Dance

Movement and Dance can be practised in a way that is therapeutic, physically and emotionally.

Two practitioners are:

Deborah Bailey, c/o 83, University St., Belfast BT7 1HP. Tel. 0232-242910;
Joan Davis, The Studio, rear 330 Harolds Cross Road, Dublin 6. Tel. 01-909118.
A variety of classes including the following :
Moving Experience — a combination of voice and movement.
Shape up and Stretch — Physicality, Fitness and Fun.
Right Brain/Left Brain Dancing.
Vibrating Vocals — breath control, voice work and improvisation.
Dance Free — Dancing for fun.

List of Practitioners of Ki Massage

All the following are members of the Irish Health Culture Association which governs Ki Massage Therapy. Costs are £10 (half hour) or £16 (one hour) with reduction for courses of treatment.

Carlow:
Ben Donnelly MIHCA, 1 Laurel Park, Pollerton, Carlow; Josephine Donnelly MIHCA, 1 Laurel Pk., Pollerton, Carlow.
Cork:
Jeremiah O'Sullivan MIHCA, 19 Shandon Street, Cork. Tel. 963191 (11-2pm); Francoise Quiniou MIHCA, 7 Church St., Off Shandon St., Cork; Michael Clair MIHCA, 54 Silverdale Ave., Ballinlough, Co. Cork. Tel. 021-291900; Phil O'Brien MIHCA, 52 Cahergal Lawn, Ballyhooley Rd., Cork. Tel. 021-506397; Joan Galvin MIHCA, 27 Melbourne Road, Bishopstown, Co. Cork. Tel. 021-544380; Patrick Crowe MIHCA, Ballynaneening, Fountainstown, Co. Cork. Tel. 021-831742; Nancy Finucane MIHCA, Ballynaneening, Fountainstown, Co. Cork. Tel. 021-831742; Nuala O'Sullivan MIHCA, Vermont, Hartlands Ave., Cork. Tel. 021-964415; Teresa Foley MIHCA, 6 Rockgrove Tce., Lr. Glanmire Rd., Cork. Tel. 021-50937.
Kerry:
Helen Higgins MIHCA, Ballineetig, Dingle, Co. Kerry. Tel. 066-51213; David Sankar MIHCA, 5 Urban Tce., Boherbee, Tralee, Co. Kerry. Tel. 066-24035.
Kildare:
Mildred Hegarty MIHCA, 88 Glendale Est., Leixlip, Co. Kildare. Tel. 242308; Noel Donagher MIHCA, 1411 St. Evan's Park, Monasterevin, Co. Kildare. Tel. 045-41203.
Kilkenny:
Sean Kelly MIHCA, Leggettsrath, Dublin Road, Kilkenny. Tel. 056-22462.
Limerick:
Helen Whelehan MIHCA, Apt B4, Wellesley Ct., Limerick. Tel. 061-54473; Marie Costelloe MIHCA, 1 Clare View Tce., Sth. Circular Rd., Limerick. Tel. 061-310156.

Louth:
Patrick Lee MIHCA, 196 Point Rd., Dundalk, Co. Louth. Tel:. 042-31866; Edward Stewart MIHCA, Ammies, Kilcurry, Dundalk, Co. Louth. Tel. 042-39908.
Meath:
Mary Cromwell MIHCA, 2 Greenfield Grove, Ashbourne, Co. Meath. Tel. 350581; Plunkett Cromwell MIHCA, 2 Greenfield Grove, Ashbourne, Co. Meath. Tel. 350581.
Monaghan:
Dolores Farrell MIHCA, 50 Highfield, Carrickmacross, Co. Monaghan. Tel. 04-63092; Tom Marron MIHCA, 1 Mullinery, Carrickmacross, Co. Monaghan; Liam Thornton MIHCA, Magheraboy, Carrickmacross, Co. Monaghan. Tel. 042-61884; Noreen Townshend MIHCA, Aghalile Road, Carrickmacross, Co. Monaghan. Tel. 042-61788.
Offaly:
Patricia Hoedt MIHCA, 22 Arden Vale, Tullamore, Co. Offaly. Tel. 0506-21084.
Tipperary:
Peggy Quirke MIHCA, Ballyea, Cahir, Co. Tipperary. Tel. 052-41962.
Waterford:
Rena Stokes MIHCA, 12 Upr. Johnstown, Ballytruckle Rd., Waterford. Tel. 051-70277; Monica Ryan MIHCA, 3 Debbyn St., Passage East, Co. Waterford. Tel 051-81475.
Wicklow:
Hanoria Ginty MIHCA, Ard na Greine, Monastery Road, Enniskerry, Co. Wicklow. Tel. 860574; Alex Warren MIHCA, 49 Heather Vue, Greystones, Co. Wicklow. Tel. 877763; Marie Warren MIHCA, 49 Heather Vue, Greystones, Co. Wicklow. Tel. 877763.
Dublin County — South & West:
James Fitzgerald MIHCA, 57 Cherbury Ct., Booterstown Ave., Blackrock, Co. Dublin. Tel. 885777; Jonathan Freestone MIHCA, 12 Grange Tce., Deansgrange Rd., Blackrock, Co. Dublin. Tel. 892694, 893955w; Sheila Hennessy MIHCA, 40 Grove Ave., Blackrock, Co. Dublin, 886201; Elinor Hickey MIHCA, 2 Glenomena Grove, Blackrock, Co. Dublin. Tel. 691844; Susan Kiernan MIHCA, 13 Villa Nova, Mt. Merrion Ave., Blackrock, Co. Dublin. Tel. 831981; John Clarke MIHCA, 15 Clarinda Pk. West, Dun Laoghaire, Co. Dublin. Tel. 841860; Katina MacCarthy MIHCA, 34 Sefton, Rochestown Ave., Dun Laoghaire, Co. Dublin. Tel. 859966; Christine Kelly MIHCA, 32 Beechwood Lawns, Killiney, Co. Dublin. Tel. 851667; Mairead Maas MIHCA, 19 Parc na Silla Road, Loughlinstown, Co. Dublin; Hazel Lidstone MIHCA MIHCA, 77 Monkstown Ave., Monkstown, Co. Dublin. Tel. 800817; Mary O'Sullivan MIHCA, 53 Cherrygarth, Mount Merrion, Co. Dublin. Tel. 884475; Marie Keenan MIHCA, 13 Corbawn Drive, Shankhill, Co. Dublin; Brid Henderson MIHCA, 13 Rockwood Park, Bray Rd., Stillorgan, Co. Dublin. Tel. 885833; Frances Moore MIHCA, 13 Roselawn, Ballydowd, Lucan, Co. Dublin. Tel. 281599.
Dublin 2:
Mark Ross MIHCA, 52 South King St., Dublin 2. Tel. 904282.
Dublin 4:
Catherina Hughes MIHCA, 68 Merrion Road, Dublin 4. Tel. 680416; Vivienne Tobin MIHCA, 92 Wilfield Road, Dublin 4. Tel. 838550; Ephrem Santiago MIHCA, 45 Wellington Rd., Ballsbridge, Dublin 4. Tel. 685914; Edmund Wall MIHCA, 22 Shelbourne Road, Ballsbridge, Dublin 4. Tel. 603876; Dora Cronin

MIHCA, 14 Rowan House, Mespil Est., Sussex Road, Dublin 4. Tel. 606386.

Dublin 6:
Caitriona Nic Ghiollaphadraig MIHCA, 23 Terenure Park, Dublin 6. Tel. 363412; James Quirke MIHCA, Brenda Hyland Clinic, 53 Ranelagh Villa, Dublin 6. Tel. 978350; Margaret Furlong MIHCA, 8 Parkview Ave., Harolds Cross, Dublin 6. Tel. 985512; Paul Hynes MIHCA, 50 Annavilla Rd., Ranelagh, Dublin 6. Tel. 963523; Maureen Travers MIHCA, 6 Hillcourt, Highfield Rd., Rathgar, Dublin 6; Mary Doyle MIHCA, 10 Kilcross, Seven Oaks, Rathmines, Dublin 6. Tel. 973853; Rosaleen Durkin MIHCA, 2 Labas Tce., Leinster Rd. West, Rathmines, Dublin 6. Tel. 979601; James Kelly MIHCA, 2 Grosvenor Square, Rathmines, Dublin 6. Tel. 973580; Norah Healy MIHCA, 6 Corrib Road, Terenure, Dublin 6. Tel. 904085.

Dublin 8:
Noreen Farell MIHCA, Basement Studio, 54 Synge St., Dublin 8. Tel. 784945; Patricia McKenna MIHCA, 2 Bloomfield Ave., Sth. Circular Rd., Dublin 8. Tel. 543319.

Dublin 10:
Eugene Traynor MIHCA, 31 Claddagh Rd., Ballyfermot, Dublin 10. Tel. 744548, 269383; Gerard Eagers MIHCA, 84 Kylemore Drive, Ballyfermot, Dublin 10. Tel. 269419.

Dublin 12:
Theresa O'Brien MIHCA, 133 Kimmage Rd. West, Dublin 12; Irene Jordan MIHCA, 51 Galtymore Close, Drimnagh, Dublin 12. Tel. 557440; Marie Brennan MIHCA, 18 Tonduff Close, Green Park, Walkinstown, Dublin 12. Tel. 513159; Patricia Cloughley MIHCA, 149 St. Peter's Rd., Walkinstown, Dublin 12. Tel. 509813.

Dublin 14:
Philip O'Connor MIHCA, 39 Rosemount Est., Dundrum, Dublin 14. Tel. 986790; Elizabeth Homan MIHCA, 6 Orchardstown Ave., Rathfarnham, Dublin 14. Tel. 943103.

Dublin 16:
Brendan Redmond MIHCA, 58 Darglewood, Knocklyon, Dublin 16. Tel. 944822; Phil Moloney MIHCA, 27 Glenvara Pk., Ballycullen Rd., Templeogue, Dublin 16. Tel. 942178.

Dublin 20:
Alan McNamara MIHCA, Stewarts Sports Centre, Palmerstown, Dublin 20. Tel. 269869w, 302312h.

Dublin 22:
Anne Nicholl MIHCA, 70 Floraville Ave., Clondalkin, Dublin 22. Tel. 591567.

Dublin County — North:
Muriel F. Neville MIHCA, 108 Hampton Cove, Balbriggan, Co. Dublin. Tel. 411342; Anne Kirwan RGN MIHCA, Corduff, Lusk, Co. Dublin; Brian Cavanagh MIHCA, O'Hanlon's Lane, Dublin Road, Malahide, Co. Dublin. Tel. 453394; Patricia May MIHCA, 90 Carrickhill Rise, Portmarnock, Co. Dublin. Tel. 461404; Siobhan Murphy-O'Hara MIHCA, 27 The Cairn, Rush, Co. Dublin. Tel. 438545; Peig Keane MIHCA, 19 Selskar Rise, Town Park, Skerries, Co. Dublin. Tel. 490020; Pauline Delaney MIHCA, 32 Ashley Ave., Malahide Road, Swords, Co. Dublin. Tel. 402071; Anne Kinsella MIHCA, 10 Chapel Lane, Swords, Co. Dublin; Donal O hObain MIHCA, 29 Forest Boulevard, River Valley, Swords, Co. Dublin. Tel. 405540.

Dublin 3:
Jacqueline Duffy MIHCA, 3 Inverness Road, Fairview, Dublin 3. Tel. 372825.

Dublin 5:
Vivienne Murphy MIHCA, 57 Brookwood Ave., Dublin 5. Tel. 311474; Bridin Nic Ionnraic MIHCA, 149 Brookwood Ave., Artane, Dublin 5. Tel. 301551h, 778060 ex430w; Pat Lynch MIHCA, 96 Abbeyfield, Killester, Dublin 5. Tel. 319754; Teresa Marren RGN MIHCA, 11 Glenayle Road, Cameron Est., Raheny, Dublin 5. Tel. 480736; Madeleine Monks MIHCA, 14 St. Assams Park, Raheny, Dublin 5.

Dublin 7:
Moya Connelly RGN RM MIHCA, 363 Navan Rd., Dublin 7. Tel. 382547; Rose Coyle MIHCA, 32 St. Ignatius Rd., Drumcondra, Dublin 7. Tel. 309253; Sheila Browne MIHCA, St. Mary's, Ashtown Cross, Navan Road, Dublin 7. Tel. 384129; Liam McDonald MIHCA, 2 St. Vincent St., Phibsboro, Dublin 7. Tel. 304584; Dympna O'Brien MIHCA, 4 Blackquiere Villas, Phisboro, Dublin 7. Tel. 300715; Aogan O'Hare MIHCA, 24 Rathdown Road, Phisboro, Dublin 7. Tel. 304816.

Dublin 9:
Maureen Carroll MIHCA, 140 Gracepark Heights, Drumcondra, Dublin 9. Tel. 379682; Frank McCabe MIHCA, 38 Dargle Road, Drumcondra, Dublin 9. Tel. 305097; Rita Kelly MIHCA, 33 Cremore Lawn, Glasnevin, Dublin 9. Tel. 346709; Celine Moore MIHCA, 11 Crestfield Road, Whitehall, Dublin 9. Tel. 374334.

Dublin 11:
Lorraine Brady-O'Leary MIHCA, 14 Cedarwood Rise, Dublin 11. Tel. 348705; Colin Smith MIHCA, 20 Glasilawn Road, Glasnevin, Dublin 11. Tel. 362361.

Dublin 15:
Adrienne Gannon CIDESCO CIBTAC MIHCA, 13 Glenville Grove, Blanchardstown, Dublin 15. Tel. 211602; Deirdre McGeough MIHCA, 2 Westway Rise, Blanchardstown, Dublin 15. Tel. 211803; Mary Dolan MIHCA, 10 Park Drive Grove, Castleknock, Dublin 15. Tel. 204029; David Fitzpatrick MIHCA, 130 Roselawn Rd., Castleknock, Dublin 15; Una McEvoy MIHCA, 10 Park Drive Grove, Castleknock, Dublin 15. Tel. 204029; Margaret Watts MIHCA, 15 Roselawn View, Castleknock, Dublin 15. Tel. 212573.

Overseas:
Daniel Butler MIHCA, 1 Mona St., Douglas, Isle of Man; Ros Scully MIHCA, c/o Jean Muldoon, 15 Tucker St., Milton, MA. 02186 U.S.A.; Mairead O'Brien MIHCA, 56 Goldsborough Close, West Lea, Swindon, SN5 7EP England; Joan Langley MIHCA, De Lairessestraat, 9, Eindhoven, The Netherlands.

Chapter Seven

REFLEXOLOGY

by Susanna Hassett and Ursula Martin

Ursula Martin *is the founder of the Reflex Zone Therapy School and of the Irish Institute of Reflexology. She practises Remedial Massage as well as Reflexology and received her training in Switzerland.*

'Foot Reflexology is based on the theory that there are areas on the feet which relate to every part of the body. The practice of Reflexology consists of working on these reflex points in a trained manner . . . and thus bringing about improvements in the functions of the various organs and systems of the body.'[1]

The first known recording of Reflexology treatment is to be found on an Egyptian tomb drawing which dates from around 2330 B.C. There is evidence to show that Reflexology was also practised in ancient Chinese, African and North American Indian civilisation.

Its revival was begun in New York in 1913 by Dr. William Fitzgerald. His work was developed further by Dr. George Starr White and Dr. Joseph Riley. Eunice Ingham, an American masseuse who worked with Dr. Riley, spent years experimenting and observing pressure massage of the feet and her work was central in establishing Reflexology as it is currently practised.

Conceptually, Reflexology divides the body into ten vertical and three horizontal zones. The feet are also divided into ten vertical and three horizontal zones. The outline of the foot is scaled to exactly the proportions of the seated human form. By means of the grid created in this fashion, the *Reflex Zone* for each organ and part of the body is located on the

---

1   *Practical Foot Reflexology* by James Morey, (Sarsinian Books, Eire,1989).

feet. The Zone for the heart is on the left foot, that for the appendix is on the right foot, the kidneys have a Zone on each foot as do the ovaries, etc.

The term *Reflex* is not used here in its strict medical meaning of a muscular contraction caused by an external stimulus and relayed by central means, such as via the spinal chord. (The knee-jerk is the most widely known instance of a reflex reaction in the strict medical sense.) Rather, it means that the feet act as a small screen that reflects the entire organism, as a reflex camera reflects the external image. It also means that there is a direct energy relationship between the Reflex Zones and the internal and external parts of the body.

The energy that flows between the feet and the rest of the body is *Life Energy*, also known as *Qi, Chi, Ki, The Vital Force* or *Universal Energy*. The channels through which Life Energy is deployed and stimulated in Reflexology are distinct from the lines of energy in Shiatsu or Acupuncture and from physiological or anatomical structures.

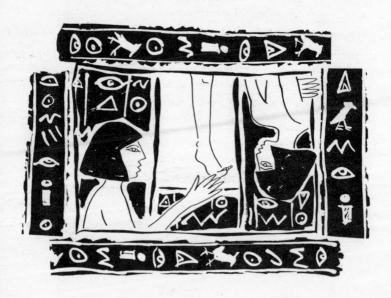

Visiting a Reflexologist

The practitioner will examine the feet, first visually and then manually in order to gain an understanding of the client's general state of health and identify any particular problems.

Visible marks such as corns, cracks, warts, athlete's foot, scars, reddening, hard skin, etc. are generally attributed to bad footwear, but may be interpreted quite differently by the Reflexologist! S/he will note the Reflex Zone where any such signs are visible and check during the manual examination for any inner debility which may have predisposed them to occur just there. The form and shape of the feet are also taken into account: for example, *fallen arches* or *flat feet* can affect the reflexes to the spinal column; a *bunion* has its effects on the reflexes to the cervical spine and the thyroid gland; *hammer toes* burden all of the reflexes to the head and also to the teeth; *injuries or congestion around the ankle and heel* indicate disorders of the pelvis and hip joint. *Swollen tissues* or *pockets of fluid* are in general attributed to a disorder of the kidneys, heart or circulation.

When the visual examination is complete, the Reflexologist will begin the manual examination by exerting pressure on each Zone. When pain is felt in a Reflex Zone, it indicates a disturbance in the corresponding organ or part of the body. When a Zone is in good condition, no pain is felt in response to pressure.

'Pain in response to pressure is a warning signal, it is the crying out of the tissues for a free flow of energy'[2]

This method of examination is also widely used by practitioners of other healing methods for the purpose of building up a picture of the client's general health. It indicates the existence not only of serious health problems, but also tells when an organ is stressed — pain will be felt in response to pressure on the Reflex Zone before the condition deteriorates to the point where the organ itself is showing symptoms. For example, the effects of an unhealthy diet on the eliminatory, excretory or circulatory systems can be detected before longterm damage to the organs themselves is evident.

2 *Reflexology*, a paper by Ursula Martin.

Following this examination, the Reflexologist will massage both feet, stimulating the free flow of energy throughout the body. Reflex Zone massage is pleasant and relaxing — it doesn't even tickle when the body is relatively healthy, but can be quite painful on those areas where there is a blockage or an accumulation of waste matter. After a treatment, the sensation is of ease, not just to the feet which tingle and glow, but to the whole body. However, one may experience an initial worsening of the presenting condition before an improvement takes place. Other common reactions are an alleviation of any pain and a marked increase in kidney activity as toxins which have been stirred up by the treatment are eliminated. Women whose menstrual cycle has been irregular may experience a fuller period than usual soon after a good Reflexology treatment. The number and frequency of treatments required varies according to the seriousness of the condition and the length of time it has been there.

Reflexology is an excellent remedy for symptoms such as headaches, sinus troubles, catarrh, insomnia, stress, bad circulation, period problems, constipation, lack of energy, muscular problems, etc. It does have its limits and is contra-indicated in the following cases : acute infectious fevers and diseases; acute inflammation of venous and lymphatic systems; deep vein thrombosis; conditions where surgery is indicated; gangrene and extensive mycotic infections of the feet; unstable pregnancies; osteoporosis and decalcification resulting from accidents leading to poor healing or malunion of bone, and possible decalcification resulting from tumours.

In civilisations based on the extended family or tribe, Reflexology was very widely practised as a Folk Medicine. It seems that it is enjoying a revival of its status as a Folk Medicine in Ireland, judging at least by the number of people who have completed courses in Reflexology but who use their skill among family and friends, not wishing to be listed here as practitioners!

In Twentieth Century industrial (or post-industrial) society, Reflexology is fast becoming a popular means of health maintenance, alleviating physical stress from whatever source before serious conditions develop. Also, where external factors are gradually contributing to the development of ill-health, Reflexology will give an early warning and allow preventative steps to be taken.

Reflexologists

There are slight variations in the methods of Reflexology practised in Ireland, represented by the different professional groupings that exist. Recently a Council including all of the bodies listed below has been formed. The Council is working hard toward the standardisation of the teaching and practice of Reflexology in Ireland.

List of Practitioners

The Society of Reflexologists of Ireland (SRI)

The SRI is a professional body of Reflexologists. Its objects include:

— The promotion of an approved programme of professional education designed to improve the standards of the practice of Reflexology for the benefit of the general public and the members of the profession.

— To promote the establishment of ethical and professional standards for the practice of Reflexology for the benefit of the general public and the members of the profession.

— To promote the support and encouragement of research applicable to Reflexology and its practice.

— To promote the establishment and maintenance of a programme to inform the general public of the benefits of Reflexology and of the requirements for the ethical practice thereof.

SRI Members

Armagh:
Eileen Kingham, 51, Salisbury Ave., Belfast BT15 5DZ. Tel. Belfast 778686; Also 35, St. James Park, Belfast BT12.

Carlow:
Maura Mahon, Springfield, Bennykerry, Carlow. Tel. 0503-31381.

Cavan:
Catherine Blake, Main St., Kingscourt, Co. Cavan. Tel. 042-67130; Maureen Campbell, Coclea, Kingscourt, Co. Cavan; Mae Ferguson, Poles, Co. Cavan. Tel. 049-36294; Mary Fitzsimons, Derryliff, Ballyconnell, Co. Cavan. Tel. 049-26161.

Clare:
Annette Gardiner, Dun Mhuire, 14 Kincora Park, Ennis, Co. Clare. Tel. 065-

21557; Imelda Moore, O'Deas Road, Kilrush, Co. Clare. Tel. 065-51223; Paul O'Brien, Barrtra, Lahinch, Co. Clare. Tel.065-81280.

Cork:

Deirdre Buckley, 36, Melbourne Road, Bishopstown, Cork. Tel. 021-545351; Jerry Longfield, The Twaites, Croaghta Park, Glasheen, Cork. Tel. 021-964776; Mark Longfield, The Twaites, Croaghta Park, Glasheen, Cork. Tel. 021-964776; J. McCabe, 87 Shamrock Drive, Muskerry Estate, Ballincollig, Cork; Elizabeth McCarthy, Padre Pio Villa, Glenabo, Fermoy, Co. Cork. Tel. 025-32473; Peter O'Donoghue, Ballymartin, Dungourney, Co. Cork. Tel. 021-668487; also Natural Healing Centre, The Twaites, Glasheen, Cork Tel. 021-964776*; Lilly O'Neill, Notre Dame, 3, Trahy Road, Togher, Cork. Tel. 021-311358; Catherine Quarry, The Manse, Ardbrack, Kinsale, Co. Cork. Tel. 021-772489.

Dublin:

Marcella Archbold, 53 Main Street, Rush, Co. Dublin Tel. 01-437529; Marie Bergin, 6, Beechpark Grove. Foxrock, Dublin 18. Tel. 01-893629; Gloria Browne, 13 Martin Grove, Blackhorse Avenue, Navan Road, Dublin 7. Tel. 01-383459; also, 7, The Drive, Kingswood Heights, Tallaght, Dublin 24. Tel. 01-522722; Marie Cleary, 174, North Rd., Finglas, Dublin 11. Tel. 01-342365; Sheila Davey, 47, Kenilworth Pk., Harolds Cross, Dublin 6. Tel. 01-976754; Bridget Doris, 39, Grove Ave., Blackrock, Co. Dublin. Tel. 01-881984; Joy Eager, 44, Woodlands Ave., Dun Laoire, Dublin. Tel. 01-859978; Olive Gentleman, 2, Laurel Park, Clondalkin, Dublin 22. Tel. 01-592460 (see also *Acupuncture*); Dympna Hall, 8, Hermitage View, Rathfarnham, Dublin 16. Tel. 01-945601; Joan Hegarty, 37, Kenure Park, Rush, Co. Dublin. Tel. 01-437529; also 53, Main St., Rush, Co. Dublin; Mary Hendron, 76, Leinster Road, Rathmines, Dublin 6. Tel. 01-967543; Sr. Attracta Kavanagh, Convent of Mercy, Beaumont, Dublin 9; Peig Keane, 19, Selskar Rise, Townpark, Skerries, Co. Dublin Tel. 01-490020; Madeline Leahy, 64, Errigal Road, Drimnagh, Dublin 12. Tel. 01-553360; Mary Moran, 69, Morehampton Rd., Donnybrook, Dublin 4. Tel. 01-944111/602298; Edith Moran, 1 Homefarm Road, Drumcondra, Dublin 9; Eileen McBarron, 1, St. Heliers Copse, Stillorgan Pk., Blackrock, Co. Dublin. Tel. 01-832611; Ann O' Dwyer, 54, Main St., Rush, Co. Dublin. Tel. 01-437176; Maeve O' Neill, 25, Monastery Crescent, Clondalkin, Dublin 22. Tel. 01-591038; Irene Ann Power, 15, Kenilworth Road, Rathgar, Dublin 6. Tel. 01-974596; Christina Russell, 25, Navan Road, Castleknock, Dublin 15. Tel. 01-213538; Rosemary Skinner, 123, Lr. Kilmacud Rd., Stillorgan, Co. Dublin. Tel. 01-884925; Mary Stefanazzi, 101, Huntstown

Wood, Mulhuddart, Dublin 15. Tel. 01-214772; also : 8, Clontarf Rd., Clontarf, Dublin 3; Joy Stone, 128, Meadow Grove, Dundrum, Dublin 16. Tel. 01-988186; also Belgrave Medical Centre, Ranelagh, Dublin 6; Mary Walsh, 60, Culmore Road, Palmerstown, Dublin 20. Tel. 01-553360; also 64, Errigal Road, Drimnagh, Dublin 12; Sr. Bregia Whelan, Convent of Mercy, Beaumont, Dublin 9; Drusilla Wynne, 30, Cross Ave., Dun Laoire, Co. Dublin. Tel. 01-800652.

Galway:
Sr. Emilian Danaher, 18, Waterside, Woodquay, Galway. Tel. 091-64776; Elizabeth Glynn, Scothill, Kilconnell, Ballinasloe, Co. Galway. Tel. 091-86666; Myriam Keaveny, 65, Tirellan Heights, Headford Rd., Co. Galway. Tel. 091-68201; Marie Therese Shelly, 51, Clybaun Heights, Knocknacarra, Galway. Tel. 091-24976.

Kerry:
Patrick Brosnan, Tubridmore, Ardfert, Co. Kerry.

Kildare:
Kay Murphy, The Paddocks, Naas, Co. Kildare. Tel.045-66531; Eileen Ryan, Convent of Mercy, Athy, Co. Kildare. Tel.0507-31361.

Limerick:
Sr. Anna Danaher, St. Johns Hospital, Limerick. Tel.061-45822.

Louth:
Geri Halpin, Mill House, Mill Lane, Drogheda, Co. Louth. Tel.041-33565; Roisin Carroll, Golf Links, Blackrock, Dundalk, Co. Louth. Tel. 042-21668; Ann Matthews, 1, St. Theresa's Tce., Scarlet St., Drogheda, Co. Louth. Tel. 041-33355.

Mayo:
Martina Barrett, 20, Pontoon Drive, Castlebar, Co. Mayo. Tel. 094-23161; Maureen Connolly, Ballinavode, Belmullet, Co. Mayo. Tel. 097-81258.

Meath:
Loretta Martin, Lambay, Kilbride, Trim, Co. Meath. Tel. 046-32486; Rose Rispin, Grange, Bohermeen, Navan, Co. Meath. Tel. 046-21563*.

Monaghan:
Mary Carroll, Tyraverty, Scotstown, Co. Monaghan. Tel. 047-89574; also : 26 Market St., Monaghan; Mary Keegan, Riverview, Carrickmacross, Co. Monaghan. Tel. 042-61475; Pauline O'Hagan, Derryolam, Carrickmacross, Co. Monaghan. Tel.042-61904.

Roscommon:
Sr. Brid McLoughlin, Convent of Mercy, Castlerea, Co. Roscommon. Tel. 0907-20127.

Tipperary:
Moyra Hennessy, Rosemary Street, Roscrea, Co. Tipperary. Tel. 0505-22192; Catherine Shelley, Seskin, Kilsheelin, Co. Tipperary. Tel.052-33115*; Sheila Tracy, Lower Main Street, Cloughjordan, Co. Tipperary. Tel. 0505-42253*.

Wexford:
Anne Bolger, St. Anthony's, Castlehill, Enniscorthy, Co. Wexford. Tel. 054-35555; also 2, Church St., Enniscorthy, Co. Wexford. Tel. 054-33192; Kate Murphy, Arnold House, Enniscorthy, Co. Wexford. Tel. 054-33484; Anthony Larkin, 51, Parkfield, New Ross, Co. Wexford. Tel. 051-22209*.

Wicklow:
Marie Boyle, Altona, Seafront, Bray, Co. Wicklow. Tel. 01-861408.

SRI Approved Schools of Reflexology

The Churchill Centre
Rose Rispin, Grange, Bohermeen, Navan, Co. Meath. Tel. 046-21563.
The Holistic School of Reflexology
Olive Gentleman, 2, Laurel Park, Clondalkin, Dublin 22. Tel. 01-592460; Mary Stefanazzi, 101, Huntstown Wood, Mulhuddart, Dublin 15. Tel. 01-214772.
The Largar College of Reflexology
Annette Gardiner, Dun Mhuire, 14, Kincora Park, Ennis, Co. Clare. Tel. 065-21557; Anthony Larkin, 41, Parkfield, New Ross, Co. Wexford. Tel. 051-22209.
The Natural Healing Centre
Jeremiah Longfield, The Twaites, Croaghta Park, Glasheen Road, Cork. Tel. 021-964776; Peter O'Donoghue, Ballymartin, Dungourney, Co. Cork. Tel. 021-668487.
The Irish Institute of Health and Healing
Maureen Connolly, Ballinavode, Belmullet, Co. Mayo. Tel. 097-81258; Mary Therese Shelley, 51, Aybawn Heights, Knocknacarra, Galway. Tel. 091-24976; Also relaxation and counselling to individuals, couples and groups.

*Additional information on Reflexology is available from Committee Members of the Society of Reflexologists, who are noted on the above list by the inclusion of the symbol * after the telephone number.

The Irish Institute of Reflexology (IIR)

The Irish Institute of Reflexology was founded in conjunction with the Reflex Zone Therapy School in 1986. The School offers practitioners diploma courses and post-graduate courses. The Institute is a practitioners' association, providing insurance for its full-time practising members and aiming to promote Reflexology. It is open to all practitioners to apply for membership. Further information is available from:
Ursula Martin, 49, Rockville Crescent, Blackrock, Co. Dublin Tel. 01-883093.

IIR Members

Antrim:
Eileen M. Bailie, 10, Cairnshill Crescent, Belfast BT8 4RL, Co. Antrim. Tel. Belfast 703012; also SRN, RMN, SCN, M.Bar.; Hilary Hoare-Doherty, 22, Tonagh Park, Lisburn, BT28 1DT, Co. Antrim. Tel. Lisburn 678611; Maureen Alison Hope-Duncan, 53, Park Rd., Belfast BT7 1FX, Co. Antrim. Tel. Belfast 691344; Eileen Kingham, 51, Salisbury Ave., Antrim Rd., Belfast BT15 5DU, Co. Antrim; Hella O'Dwyer, 3, Ferndale, Harmony Heights, Lisburn, BT274 HQ Co. Antrim; Carole Wray, 34, Lucerne Pds., Belfast BT9 5FT, Co. Antrim. Tel. Belfast 669913.
Armagh:
Deirdre Mc Kiernan, 2, Old Mill, Tandragee, Craigavon, BT62 2JH; Sheila Magee, 50, Antrim Rd., Lurgan Co. Armagh. Tel. Lurgan 6003.
Carlow:
Mary Kavanagh, Pollerton Beig, Carlow. Tel. 0503-41209.

Clare:
Eileen Daly, 35, Oak Park, Ennis, Co. Clare. Tel. 065-22073; Mary Ryan, 7, Springfield, Clonroadmore, Ennis, Co. Clare. Tel. 065-29817.

Cork:
Mary Carroll, 147, Green Hills Court, Sth. Douglas Rd., Cork; Dr. Jennifer Daly, 2, Nova Court, Ballea Rd., Carrigaline, Co. Cork; Deborah Ann McGrath, Riversdale House, Midleton, Co. Cork; Marian Flynn, Douglas Reflexology Clinic, Morris House, Douglas West, Cork. Tel. 021-891605/362402; Emer Mary Quain, 17, Tracton Park, Montenotte, Cork. Tel. 021-509571/985607; Sr. Noelle Ryan, Bon Secours Hospital, College Rd., Cork. Tel. 021-542807.

Down:
Ann Graham, 7,Cardy Close, Bangor BT19 1AT Tel. Bangor 458903.

Dublin:
Marlene Bean, "Charleville", Church Rd., Ballybrack, Co. Dublin. Tel. 01-852821; Anne Brennan, St. Patrick's Well, Kilternan, Co. Dublin. Tel. 01-955679; Ruth Brennan as above; Eileen Beechinor, 11 Glenageary Lodge, Arnold Grove, Glenageary, Co. Dublin. Tel. 01-858127; Breda Brennan, 64, Rathgar Road, Dublin 6; Patrick S. Coote, 37, Haddon Rd., Clontarf, Dublin 3. Tel. 01-333060; Veronica Cahill, 81, Whitehall Rd., Terenure, Dublin 12. Tel. 01-555906; Kevin Clark, 37, Dunvile Ave., Ranelagh, Dublin 6. Tel. 01-876917; also Therapeutic Massage; Terese Doran, Hackton, Castleknock, Dublin. Tel. 01-211726; Bridget Doris, 39, Grove Ave., Blackrock, Co. Dublin. Tel.01-881984; Margaret Duffy, 262 Navan Rd., Dublin 7. Tel. 01-384397; Tess Gannon, Drumgildra, Rathmore Villas, Terenure, Dublin 6. Tel. 01-904400; Pamela Gillespie, "Avalon", Stillorgan Rd., Donnybrook, Dublin 4. Tel. 01-693437; Una Hoggarth, 64, Claremont Rd., Sandymount, Dublin 4. Tel. 01-683024; June Mary Hannon, Castleknock House, Castleknock, Dublin 15. Tel. 01-201165/210776; Carmel Harrison, 5, Pembroke Rd., Ballsbridge, Dublin 4. Tel. 01-685331; Mary P. Hyland, 20, Maryfield Rd., Dublin 8. Tel. 01-532549; Peig Keane, 19, Selskar Rise, Townpark, Skerries, Co. Dublin. Tel. 01-490020; also Ki Massage; Paula Keegan, 51, Sutton Downs, Sutton, Dublin 13. Tel. 01-326010; Madeline Leahy, 64, Errigal Rd., Drimnagh, Dublin 12. Tel. 01-553360; Traudel Larkin, Rockfield House, Clonsilla, Dublin 15. Tel. 01-213647; Margaret Leonard, 4, Green Lawns, Skerries, Co. Dublin; Valerie Lynch, 82, Templeville Dr., Templeogue, Dublin 6; Odile Lynch, as above; Maeve Madden, 8, Glandore Rd., Griffith Ave., Dublin 9. Tel. 01-378311; Ursula Martin, 49, Rockville Crescent, Blackrock, Co. Dublin. Tel. 01-883093; also Remedial Massage; Stanley Moore, Barnaby Dun, Cherrywood Rd., Loughlinstown, Co. Dublin. Tel. 01-822948; Teresa Mc Court, 6, Nutgrove Pk., Clonskea, Dublin 14. Tel. 01-694522; Lynda McCool, 24 College Cresc., Terenure, Dublin 6. Tel. 01-901935; Dr. Maeve McGrath, 12, Dunmore Pk., Ballymount, Dublin 24. Tel. 01-511453; Also General Practice, Relaxation, Psychotherapy, St. Paul's Ministry of Divine Healing on Mondays at 8.30pm.; Bernie McNamara, 100 Grange Rd., Baldoyle, Dublin 13. Tel. 01-324235; Patricia McKee, 58, Thormanby Rd., Howth, Co. Dublin. Tel. 01-324713; Ann Noonan, "Westwood", 2, Churchview Rd., Killiney, Co. Dublin. Tel. 01-854144; Terese O'Brien, 45 Bulfin Rd., Dublin 8. Tel. 01-540709; Ruth O'Reilly, 33, The Rise, Kingswood Heights, Knogswood, Dublin 24. Tel. 01-97098; Phil O'Doherty, 8, Cliffort Ave., Malahide, Co. Dublin. Tel. 01-450642; Deirdre O'Connell, 6, Roebuck Rd., Clonskeagh, Co. Dublin. Tel. 01-697320; Margaret Philbin, 57, Killakee View, Firhouse, Co. Dublin. Tel. 01-510072; Mary Power, 17, Watermill Lane, Raheny, Dublin 5. Tel. 01-310467; Sarah Power, 411,

Whitehall Rd., Terenure Dublin 12; Maura Purcell, 32, Cypress Grove South, Templeogue, Dublin 6; Jimmy Quirke, 26, Belmont Ave., Donnybrook, Dublin 4. Tel. 01-713136/696127; Cecilia Slevin, 160, Corrib Rd., Terenure, Dublin 6. Tel. 01-900195; Anne South, Ken Park, Lucan, Dublin. Tel. 01-280105; Joy Stone, 128 Meadow Grove, Dundrum, Dublin 16. Tel. 01-988168; Rita Shannon, 52, Kimmage Rd. West., Terenure, Dublin 6. Tel. 01-555267; Mary Walsh, 64, Errigal Rd., Drimnagh, Dublin. Tel. 01-553360(9-12am); Jennifer Ward, 4, Whitethorn Lodge, Rathfarnham, Dublin 14. Tel. 01-904432.

Galway:
Marian Bourke, 202, Castlelawn Heights. Headford Rd., Galway. Tel. 091-66251; also R.P.N., R.S.N., M.E.Dip.; Margaret Gordon, Bothar Bui, Carraroe, Connemara, Co. Galway. Tel. 091-95217/95202.

Kerry:
Maura Galvin, Feacle, Ballyferriter, Co. Kerry.

Kildare:
Angela Abbey, 1, Temple Mills, Celbridge, Co. Kildare. Tel. 01-288742; Elizabeth Anne Aspell, St. Rita's, Blackmiller Hill, Kildare; Also SRN; Dolores Gavin, 10, West House, The Grove, Celbridge, Co. Kildare. Tel. 01-271892; Edwina Hanley, "Hazeldene", Green Rd., Kildare. Tel. 045-22192; Kay Murphy, 64, The Paddocks, Naas, Co. Kildare. Tel. 045-66531; Sr. Eileen Ryan, Convent of Mercy, Athy, Co. Kildare. Tel. 0507-31361; Also Holistic Massage. Yvonne Tone, 644, River Forest, Leixlip, Co. Kildare. Tel. 01-244133.

Leitrim:
Rhona Conlon, Church St., Ballinamore, Co. Leitrim.

Limerick:
Sara Finley, 2, Perry Sq., Limerick. Tel. 061-45351/45255; Kathleen O'Connor, "St. Joseph's", Cloncrippo, Kilmallock, Co. Limerick.

Longford:
Josephine McGovern-Matthews, Credit Union House, Market St., Granard, Co. Longford. Tel. 043-86114.

Louth:
Fidelma Arthur, Doylesfort Rd., Dundalk, Co. Louth. Tel. 042-38919.

Mayo:
Martina Barrett, 20, Pontoon Drive, Castlebar, Co. Mayo. Tel. 094-23161; Emer Gaffney, Cloona Health Centre, Westport, Co. Mayo. Tel. 098-25827/66150; Josephine Sweeney, Knockmore, Ballina, Co. Mayo. Tel. 094-58131.

Meath:
Sylvia Caffrey, Baltrasna Lane, Ashbourne, Co. Meath. Tel. 01-350551; Also Ki Massage; Margaret Corr, Grange Bective, Navan, Co. Meath. Tel. 046-29456; Mary Hutton, 10, St. Peter's Park, Dun Boyne, Co. Meath. Tel. 01-255386/255250; Also a Herbalist in Sean Boylan's practice; Arthur Rafferty, Milltown, Ashbourne, Co. Meath.

Monaghan:
Mary Fennell, Image Beauty Care, Shopping Centre, Carrickmacross, Co. Monaghan. Tel. 042-61312; Also Aromatherapy massage; Mary Keegan, "Riverview", Carrickmacross, Co. Monaghan. Tel. 042-61475.

Tipperary:
Moyra Hennessy, Rosemary St., Roscrea, Co. Tipperary. Tel. 0505-22192; Diana Moynan, Glenville, Hoganspass, Nenagh,Co. Tipperary. Tel. 067-31456; Tim McSherry, Nenagh Rd., Borrisaleigh, Co. Tipperary.

Waterford:
Ruth Gamble, Cullinagh House, Kilmeaden, Co. Waterford.

Wexford:
Ann T. Bolger, "St. Anthony's", Castle Hill, Enniscorthy, Co. Wexford.
Wicklow:
Aine Bailey, 169 Redford Pk., Greystones, Co. Wicklow. Tel. 01-877369; Kevin Clark, "Willowgrove", Delgany, Co. Wicklow. Tel. 01-876917; Also Therapeutic Massage; Teresa O'Connor, 4, Eglinton Rd., Bray, Co. Wicklow.

The Chrysalis Holistic Centre, 62, Burn Rd., Cookstown, Co. Tyrone. Tel. Cookstown 62090; Phyllida Templeton runs the Chrysalis Centre. She practices and teaches Reflexology and Yoga as well as working in Meta-Physical Counselling, Yoga Therapy, Externalization work, Healing the hurt child; She is a Montessori Directoress, a Humanistic Psychologist, with Diplomas in Yoga and Naturopathy and is a facilitator with Dr. Elizabeth Kubler-Ross workshops.

Graduates of the Chrysalis Holistic Centre
Derry:
Bernie Donnelly, Meadow Bank, Magharefelt, Co. Derry.
Donegal:
Eileen Brown, Rectory Lane, Ketterkenny, Co. Donegal; Mary Kelly, The Bridge, Ramelton, Co. Donegal; Also teaches Yoga; Janet Loughrey, Kerrykeel, Co.Donegal; Ann Malone, Bonany, Letterkenny, Co. Donegal; Ann Meade, The Diamond, Lifford, Co. Donegal. Tel. 074-41535; Sheila Meehan, "Ard Erin", Moville, Co. Donegal; Eilish McCarroll, The Glebe, Donegal Town. Tel. 073-22144; Catherine McCrory, "Woodlands", Letterkenny, Co. Donegal; Fiona McDwyer, "Hazelwood", Kilraine, Glenties, Co. Donegal; Muriel McElkinney, Gortnavern, Letterkenny, Co. Donegal; Carry McGahern, Glencush, Ballindrait, Lifford, Co. Donegal; Maura McHugh, Maura's Beauty Salon, Port Rd., Letterkenny, Co. Donegal. Tel. 074-24624; also teaches Yoga; Rose O'Donnell, "Ard Alainn", Ballintra, Aranmore Islands, Letterkenny, Co. Donegal; Brenda O'Neill, 36, Lr. Main St., Letterkenny, Co. Donegal; Heather Scott, 9, Beechgrove Ave., Letterkenny, Co. Donegal; Jennifer Taylor, Carrickshandrum, Killygordon, Co. Donegal; Also teaches Yoga.
Leitrim:
Margaret Cosgrove, Ballinagar, Drumahair, Co. Leitrim. Tel. 64236.
Sligo:
Eileen McGarry, "Brooklee", Woodville Rd., Sligo. Tel. 071-62885.

Independent Practitioners

The Reflexology Clinic, 81-82, Gt. William O'Brien St., Cork. Tel. 021-372400/500218; James and Stephanie Morey – Reflexology – Auriculo Therapy and Chiropody; James Morey is the author of *'Practical Foot Reflexology'*, (Sarsinian Press).
Patricia Swann, Meitheal Centre, Inch Island, Co. Donegal. Tel. 077-60323. Reflexology in conjunction with the Bach Flower Remedies. Linda Hassett, 12 Belvedere Rd., Dublin 1. Tel. 01-599394.

Northern Ireland Practitioners

Eilish Corrigan, Mount Royal, 5, Victoria Rd., Dungannon. Tel. Dungannon 22106; James Courtney, 35, Wynchurch Park, Belfast BT6 0JL. Tel. Belfast 645578; Elizabeth Cranston, 14, Abbey Lane, Armagh. Tel. Armagh 522132; Also at 10, Manderley Court, Portadown, Co. Armagh. Tel. Portadown 350152; Also Bach Flower Remedies and Kinesiology; Anne Hegarty, 55, Larkhill, Steelstown Rd., Derry. Tel. Derry 53118; Ann Belinda Lewis, 10, Wingrove Gdns, Belfast BT5 5NA. Tel. Belfast 653081; Olive McGarvey, 76, Strand Rd., Portstewart BT55 7LY. Tel. Portstewart 2974; Patrick McKenna, 12 & 14, Abbey Lane, Armagh. Tel. Antrim 522132; Also Bach Flower Remedies and Kinesiology; Jean McMaster, 11, Hillcrest, The Folly, Antrim BT41 1LA. Tel. Antrim 65247; Sr. Maria McNiece, Cloona House, 31, Colin Rd., Poleglass, Dunmurry. Tel. Dunmurry 626221; Sheila Nugent, 14, Central Ave., Cookstown, BT80 8AJ Tel. Cookstown 65221; Sheila Reynolds, 243, Whitepark Rd., Bushmills BT57 8SP. Tel. Bushmills 31383; also Yoga and Guest House with vegetarian wholefood cooking.

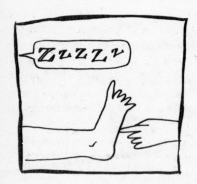

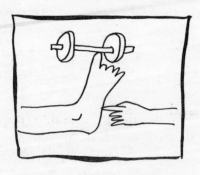

Chapter Eight

HOMEBIRTH

Women's right to control their bodies has been one of the most controversial issues in this country in the last decades. My involvement has been to campaign for free, legal and safe contraception at the time the Family Planning Bill was first mooted in 1976. Subsequently I was involved in Women's Groups of various kinds and I campaigned against the insertion of a clause into the Constitution that would give rights to the unborn foetus equal to those of its mother.

It is my view, that to become pregnant and to give birth should be a matter of joyful choice, not a burden or something to be done in order to be a real woman. Practitioners listed in this chapter, or in any part of this book, may or may not agree with these views.

A couple of years after the Abortion Referendum, I gave birth to my first child in hospital. I was nervous and tense and checked in early in the labour. It started to go wrong immediately. First of all, the nurse who booked me in insisted that my pubic hair had to be shaved. I had been assured during ante-natal classes in the same hospital that this was optional. She was quite insistent however, and said that pubic hair would add to the risk of infection . . . I knew this was rubbish, but decided to give in and save my energy for the birth itself. My heart was sinking, and my stomach turning over; I was dreading the itch as the hair grew back. I was wondering if I would have any choice during the rest of the labour. I didn't.

I wanted a natural birth. No drugs; squatting; kneeling or lying down; father present; easy on the baby; emotionally secure; the birth of a new and hopefully, free, spirit. As the cylinders of gas, masks, gowns, metal and antiseptic gradually invaded, I grew more and more tense and cervical dilation was slow. The staff were going off duty in a few hours and wanted to do me during that shift rather than switching over in the middle. As they piled on the technology, the birth slowed down and down. I grew more and more tense, and I stopped being able to feel the baby, I couldn't tell where he was, what was him or what was me. That precious contact, so strong during the last weeks of pregnancy, was gone.

During my twelve hour technological labour, four different people examined me internally, seven times, to see how far my cervix was dilated. As the baby's head crowned, I was out of my mind with pain and high with pain-killers. The Registrar produced a gleaming forceps, I yelled 'Nooooooo' and pushed, ripping my body from vagina to anus.

But the baby, every millimetre of his nine pound body, what a glorious feeling to hold him, to stroke him, to comfort each other. Oops, he's gone, time for washing him, and stitching me. 'No', I said, 'stitch me later, I want to feed him now'. They conceded. I gently took his thumb from his mouth, and stroked the side of his face so that he would turn his head, as I had seen my mother do. He looked at my nipple, opened his mouth, and he was home. Peace for ten minutes. I was amused that they covered my body before leaving the room...Stitch, stitch, I didn't even ask how many.

Three days later, I collapsed in the hospital toilet, after passing clots of blood; Uterine infection. Eight more days in

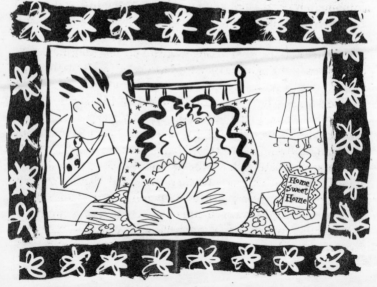

hospital, on intravenous antibiotics. When I was given a blood transfusion I broke out in a rash an hour after the blood began to transfuse and they removed it. Every time Fionn cried, I fed him. He was my lifeline, but I was also exhausted. Every time I turned over to sleep; he woke up. Every time I left the room; he cried. Every time I wanted to eat; most times anyone else touched him; he wanted me and only me. So it was for a year after. Day and night.

Political meetings — I fell asleep; At work — I was a zombie. Meeting with the Bank Manager — two nappies and a wad of wet tissue came out of my bag along with the Cash Flow projections, all stuck together with the sticky tape on the nappies. Nights out — I worried about the baby, and the babysitter, and the front of my blouses gradually moistened with milk. Housework — non-stop arguments or bad vibes. Sex — oh no, not someone else wanting a bit of me. Who am I? Where am I? Will it never end.

Well, it did, gradually. Thirteen months later, I became pregnant again. An abortion or a Home Birth were the two options I considered. Ultimately I choose the latter. Brian was born in our bedroom, one sunny August evening. The labour was powerful, it only hurt when I laughed, and only stopped while the midwife and I waited for Tommy (the childrens' father). Sarah, a friend who is an Aromatherapist, burned a combination of fragrant oils to stimulate the birth and guard against infection. We lived in a block of flats then, and as the contractions intensified, I heard a neighbour calling to her child: 'Get off that bike'. Laughing, I lost the rhythm during two contractions and Sarah magically produced oils for me to inhale. I was restored.

When Brian was born, I started to croon, I couldn't help it. My mother came on the train, bringing peace and order to the household. A lot of the children on the balcony (there were nearly thirty) were puzzled that I hadn't gone to hospital to buy my baby. One little girl stopped the doctor to ask if he'd brought him in his bag. Another suggested that he'd been wrapped up in silver paper to keep him warm. Fionn, then aged nearly two, explained that he'd come out of my tummy . . .

Aromatherapy massage the following day, for me. The doctor who I had attended throughout the pregnancy and who also attended part of the birth saw this, and to my delight he came back with Sesame oil the day after and massaged Brian, showing me how to do it. Brian breastfed 3-4 hourly, sleeping and gurgling in between. Nights were soon peaceful, sex was soon enjoyable, we caught up on the housework every so often, I prolonged my maternity leave.

Now, the feminist movement, or sections of it, are re-evaluating the campaigns of the 60s and 70s. We are dubious about the side-effects of the contraceptive pill and chemical spermicides. Having gained some ground for women in the workplace, we are looking for ways to protect women who want both to have a career and children. We fight against the feminisation of poverty, the fact that working class women are forced, through poverty, into both roles, without choice, without adequate healthcare or childcare.

Are there natural alternatives to the contraceptive pill? To travelling to England for abortions? Perhaps it is too soon for these questions, perhaps we still remember our sisters, the witches, who were burned for their wisdom.

The Hospital Birth package deal

My experience of giving birth in a hospital was one of the worst of its kind and my experience of home birth one of the best. As a result, I would not go back to hospital if I was having another baby, unless there were definite problems during pregnancy that could not be handled at a home birth. On the other hand, many women fear the prospect of giving birth without hospital expertise and equipment to hand and welcome the time in hospital as a break away from the house; isn't there a joke about having a holiday in the Maternity Ward?

However, the following aspects of the public hospital birth package deal are unacceptable to many women: there is no continuity in antenatal care — women are examined by different members of staff on virtually every antenatal visit; a check-up during pregnancy can take up to four hours, most of that time spent in queues; there are broken agreements about policy — for example whether the woman can stand or walk during labour; there are often hassles about the presence or role of fathers during the birth; there are tensions between

148

midwives and medical staff; technology is used in many cases in a way that promotes anxiety, slowing things down. Other issues arise during hospital births around the handling of the baby on birth; conflicting advice on breast-feeding; babies are stored away from the mother and sometimes fed glucose without permission; it is virtually mandatory to stay in hospital for five days after giving birth.

Irish hospitals appear to be particularly rigid, unlike other countries where there are a range of options in both hospital and home births. In Holland, for example, home birth is very widely availed of and there are 'flying squads' equipped to give fast back-up and deal with emergencies. Many English hospitals offer a range of options such as greater involvement for the father, friends or family of the woman giving birth; flexibility about discharge; greater choice as regards the use of technology and drugs during labour. In Ireland, the options are polarised, particularly for woman in public care. There is the option of the hospital birth package deal as described above or of a home birth without the type of back-up that can be necessary.

Home Birth in Ireland

Home Birth is not widely available in Ireland at present. Midwives attending Home Births must have the State qualification in midwifery and must register with the Health Board. Under The Mother and Child Scheme, they are entitled to be paid for each delivery. However, the money paid is so little and the bureaucracy involved so great, that midwives normally charge a fee.

Under the Health Boards' Scheme, they are entitled to a maximum payment of forty-odd pounds, they are obliged to see the mother and baby daily for ten days after the birth and money is deducted from the forty pounds if the mother has to go to hospital, if the midwife does not carry out so many visits, etc. etc. If they accept the Health Board's fee, they cannot make an additional charge to the client. Midwives attending Home Births can only take bookings every three to four weeks, or at longer intervals, given that babies are born when they are ready, give or take a fortnight from the predicted date. The Health Board Fee does not even cover expenses, let alone provide an income. Therefore, women, or couples, wishing to have a Home Birth are generally obliged to pay for this service.

The fees charged by the midwives listed vary according to the circumstances of the client — and indeed, according to the circumstances of the midwife. If you want a Home Birth, it is worth enquiring into the possibility of a reduced fee, or of gradual payment. And don't forget to claim the eight pound grant given by the Health Board to mothers having a Home Birth!

In addition to a midwife who attends the birth itself, it is necessary to have a doctor who will perform check-ups during the pregnancy and attend the birth. Most hospitals will not provide their services and facilities to women who intend to have a Home Birth. During my second pregnancy, my doctor and I thought it advisable to have a scan, to check on the baby's position. In order to get the scan, I had to book into the hospital in question, and endure an hour of brow-beating by a male doctor who wanted me to swear an oath there and then that I would not have a Home Birth.

The State will pay doctors for each antenatal visit by the expectant mother. A fee for the birth and any subsequent care will also be paid. There is a blatant inequality, as most doctors are men, midwives all women. Expectant mothers will go to the doctor's surgery for check-ups during surgery hours, whereas midwives have to be on-call 24 hours, must travel to the client's house, and theirs is the greater skill.

Bureaucracy aside, however, my experience was that it was wonderful to see the same person throughout a pregnancy, to get to know the people who will deliver the baby. I found it disorienting to queue in hospital and see different people every visit. Generally, doctors attending pregnancies and Home Births take a back seat during the delivery — mine said 'I'll leave that for the women, you know best' — but are there if needed. Midwives listed will supply the names of doctors who work with them for Home Births. The midwives listed below practise full-time and travel the length and breadth of the country in their work. There are other experienced midwives who take clients from time to time and who it may be possible to contact through those listed below. Having conquered all the red-tape, you will appreciate the advantages of Home Birth even more!

Midwives

Anne Kelly, 30, Brooklawn Wood, Blackrock, Co. Dublin. Tel. 01-883662; Catherine Spillane, 78, Bayside Crescent, Sutton, Co. Dublin. Tel. 01-391158; Dolores Staunton, "Khublei", Harristown, Kilcloon, Co. Meath. Tel. 01-285302; Christina Holt, The Cottage, Kilcoran, Cannon, Co. Kilkenny. Tel. 056-28216.

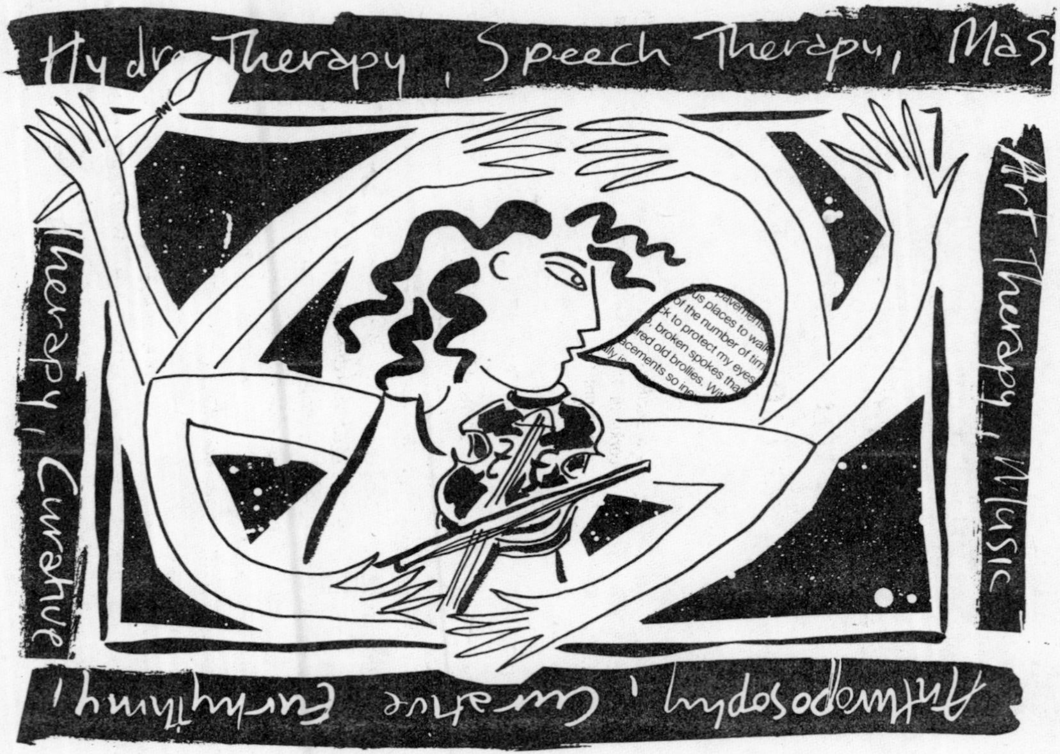
Hydro Therapy, Speech Therapy, Mas
Art Therapy, Music
Anthroposophy, Curative Eurhythmy,
Therapy, Curative

Chapter Nine

ANTHROPOSOPHY

An Extension of Medicine — Medicine based on Anthroposophy

by Dr. Maria van den Berg

Dr. Maria ven den Berg *is a Medical Doctor and doctor of Anthroposophical Medicine. Maria lives and works in the Camphill Communities in Ireland and Portugal and does not have a private practice.*

Introduction

In our time we are confronted with a great and urgent search for alternative medicine. The needs of patients are obviously not fully met by modern orthodox medicine. Thus patients, and doctors too, look for other ways of healing. Partially this arises out of the need of patients who often subconsciously feel that, though they may perhaps be cured, they are, after all, not healed by that which medicine today can offer. As a result in the last decades a wide range of different diagnostic and therapeutic methods has been re-discovered and become available. Most of them are taken from other, often past, cultures and are based on the religious and philosophical views in which these cultures are (were) rooted, (e.g. acupuncture, faith healing, aromatherapy). Others are based on the original insight individuals had (e.g. homeopathy — Hahnemann, Bach Flower remedies) or on the experiences of individuals (e.g. *iroscopy*).

Frequently alternative therapies can help, or cure. Here too, often a real healing process does not take place and a

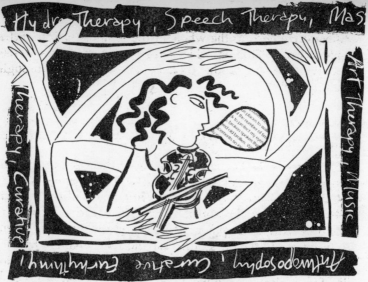

shopping around of the various alternatives starts, or one has to return over long periods for further treatment without a fundamental change in the disease condition. Something which is a basic need of modern man is not answered by these alternative ways of medicine : the possibility to learn to understand how diagnosis (*dia*: through, *gnosis*: wisdom) comes about, and how the diagnosis is related to the therapy. Other questions remain equally unanswered: why does one become ill; how is the illness related to one's life?

Some branches of alternative medicine try to meet these questions by assembling different alternative ways of diagnosis and treatments e.g. in holistic medicine. But because these different ways of diagnosis and treatment have their roots in different views of the human being it remains an attempt. One is not really able to unite these totally different views concerning the human being to the reality of the wholeness, which the human being presents. The result looks like the scattered picture of a puzzle made up out of pieces of different puzzles.

As such, modern medicine, as well as the different forms of alternative medicine can be right and helpful, when used for the right person, at the right time, in the right place and with the right consciousness. In order to be able to judge this, one requires a grounding out of which one can relate these different methods to the whole of the actual situation of the patient. This grounding, which enables judgement (diagnosis) and the findings of the therapy, can be gained through anthroposophy.

Anthroposophy — Wisdom of man

At the end of the last and beginning of this century, Rudolf Steiner (1861 — 1925) brought new perspectives to the relationships between the human spirit, soul and body; their relationship with the surrounding nature and the cosmos. and of human-development and world-development, as well as insights into the laws of karma and reincarnation. Rudolf Steiner was able to relate his research in these realms to modern scientific thinking. These insights on the one hand and the way in which one can gradually grow towards these insights, come forth out of what Rudolf Steiner called Anthroposophy — wisdom of man. In many books and lectures Rudolf Steiner has written and spoken about these aspects of human life.

Based on these insights Dr. Steiner, together with Ita Wegman, MD, initiated and developed the basic ideas and practical implications for an extension of the art of healing. Since then this has been further developed and differentiated by a growing group of doctors. This today is known as anthroposophical medicine. From the background of anthroposophy patient and doctor can, through their shared efforts, find a path to healing, to prevention of (further) disease or complications and to the meaning of illness in one's life. Though, as we know, it is not always possible to cure a disease, one can often find a different approach to it and learn to live with the illness in a positive and fruitful way. Therapies, support and treatment will help in this situation to start a healing process also where there is no cure is to be found.

Through anthroposophy one can also learn why a certain treatment helps (or not), whether orthodox or alternative, and how it works. The examples below illustrate only a fraction of the capacity of anthroposophical medicine, yet can show how with its aid one can gain insight into the relation between diagnosis and therapy.

Some basic concepts and thoughts — Spirit, Soul and Body

In general when one speaks about the human being, one often speaks about *body*, *soul* and *spirit* as three entities. What we mean by this and how they relate is often very vague to us. Rudolf Steiner defines these three realms in a very precise way, as he was able to see these realms. We too can learn to think and experience what he describes. I refer to this in the following description.

We meet, in fact, in the body of the human being the outcome, the result of the working together of four different groups of forces. As each group is an entity of forces, we can call them four different bodies. Thus we can identify:

the physical body
the etheric body
the astral body
the ego body or ego organisation.

Steiner speaks about this in his book *Theosophy*. He explains that the forces of the physical body find parallel in the mineral kingdom; the forces of the etherbody in the plant kingdom (living, growing, reproducing); and the forces of the astral-body in the animal kingdom (drives, instincts, movements). The forces of the ego-body or ego-organisation are unique to the human being and we do not share them with any other being on earth. In this way man forms, in the realm of the body, a kingdom of his own. Through the working together of these four 'bodies' our visible physical body is formed.

The interaction and relation of these bodies is different in different stages of life. In three distinct processes of metamorphosis around the seventh, fourteenth and twenty-first year a part of their forces leave their work within the visible physical body behind and turn towards serving different realms of the soul. So the same forces which first served the building up of the body can, through the process of metamorphosis, be found in the soul of the human being. Ether forces become the bearers of the thinking (this starts to happen around the seventh year); astral forces work in the feeling, (around the fourteenth year); and ego-forces work in the will of the human soul (around the twenty-first year).

Within the body and within the soul one can recognise a force which is at work, which is unique to the human being. For the body we pointed to the ego-organisation in this respect. With the help of the realm of thinking within the soul, the human being is able to form thoughts out of that which he perceives through the senses. Our Ego which is a 'drop of the Spirit' in us — can relate consciously, and therefore not only in a reactive way as the animals do, to the surrounding world.

From this one can see the concrete relationship between the body, the soul and the spirit in man and can learn to understand why psychological stress can manifest in physical illness and why physical illness influences the psyche. That this will express itself differently in different persons, (e.g. one person gets migraine, another low back pain, a third a stomach ulcer) can also become understandable, when one realises that for every individual the physical-, ether-, astral- and ego-body are differently formed and constituted.

Just as our visible physical body is different for every human being and consists of many different organs, tissues, forms, forces and processes, so also the etheric- astral- and ego- body are in themselves manifold and differentiated. Just as we need a longer and intensive study to learn to know the physical body (as is done in medical school), it also requires an intensive and long study to learn to know the other bodies. Through study, observation and exercises a doctor, who chooses to do so, can learn more and more about these subjects. In fact this is possible for everybody and it would be very helpful to learn to understand one's own and others' constitution and through this understanding become more able to prevent illness or go through illness in a meaningful way towards healing. At the beginning I referred to the relationship of the different bodies with the surrounding world; the physical body to the mineral world, the ether-body to the plant world, the astral-body to the animal world.

Through a study of nature the doctor is able to find the remedies in the surrounding world according to the diagnosis, since the same forces are at work outside in nature as within the human being.

Biography

Through the process of patient and doctor working together it is often possible to gradually find out why one falls ill at this particular age. By working together at the biography of the patient with the knowledge of the different phases of life (which can be discovered with the help of anthroposophy) it can gradually become clear what can be learned from this illness; what its true meaning is. Through this the disease does not remain a mere nuisance, but it can help one to learn more about oneself and one's purpose in life. In the same manner one can find ways to prevent illness.

These are two examples, which can give some insight as to how patient and doctor can work together with the help of anthroposophy. However it is not necessary for the patient to know about anthroposophy before consulting a doctor who works in anthroposophy.

The Practice

Since the publication of the book *Fundamentals of Therapy* written by Rudolf Steiner and Ita Wegman MD in 1925 a range of different medicines and therapies have been developed. As previously stated, the medicines used are nature-substances, which, by going through different pharmaceutical processes (e.g. rhythmical potentizing) become a healing remedy. Alongside the medicines the therapies have proven to be of great help in the healing process. At present the following therapies exist: *Nursing therapies* (care, compresses, oilings); *rhythmical massage* according to Ita Wegman; *hydrotherapy*; *curative eurythmy* (an aesthetic as well as curative dance-form); *music-therapy*; *speech-therapy*; and *art-therapy*. By the very nature of Anthroposophy it follows, that there is a continuous further research and development of these therapies. Doctors who practice this extension of medicine, have graduated in medical school and decided to go on studying in the realms described above. Conferences, courses and other post-graduate training possibilities are regularly organised to foster an ongoing developing process.

Conclusion

Many other areas are furthered and fructified by anthroposophy e.g. agriculture (bio-dynamic farming and gardening), pedagogy (the Rudolf Steiner or Waldorf pedagogy), sociology (threefold social order), curative education.

Further reading

Added is a small list of books which can be helpful to read in order to arrive at a deeper understanding of the human being and the surrounding world.

Theosophy, by Rudolf Steiner (Rudolf Steiner Press, London).
Knowledge of the Higher Worlds, by Rudolf Steiner (as above).
Health and Illness, by Rudolf Steiner (The Anthroposophic Press, Springvalley, New York).
Caring for the Sick at Home, by T.V. Bentheim, A.O. (Floris Books).
The Human Soul, by Karl Konig.(Anthroposophic Press).
Man on the Threshold, by Bernard Lievegoed (Hawthorn Press).

List of Centres

The Camphill Communities are perhaps the best known aspect of anthroposophical work in Ireland. They offer those in need of special care — children, adolescents and adults — a sheltered environment in which their educational, therapeutic and social needs can be met. A Rudolf Steiner system of general education has also developed to form the largest independent School movement in the world. There are three Steiner Schools in Ireland. There are also a number of bio-dynamic farms and a small number of practitioners of Anthroposophical Medicine. There are four Camphill Communities in the South and three in the North of Ireland.

Northern Ireland

Clanabogan Village Community, 15, Drudgeon Road, Clanabogan, Omagh, Co. Tyrone BT7B 1TJ. Tel. Omagh 41627; Farming, gardening and domestic work activities have so far been established.

Glencraig Community, Craigavad, Holywood, Co. Down BT18 ODB. Tel. Holywood 3396. Glencraig now concentrates on curative education and further education and training from pre-school until early adulthood.

Mourne Grange Village Community, Newry Road, Kilkeel, Co. Down BT34 4EX Tel. Kilkeel 62228. The community has established farms and gardens and now has workshops for pottery, woodwork, baking, laundry and domestic work. Further development in this community of 120 people will serve to emphasise its increasing maturity.

Southern Ireland

Ballytobin Community, Callan, Co. Kilkenny. Tel. 056-25114.   School, therapies and farm and garden work.

Camphill Community Dunshane, Dunshane House, Brannockstown, Co. Kildare. Tel. 045-83628/83717. A training college for adolescents in need of special education and care. Land based with craft workshops and 'Upper School' Waldorf curriculum. Duffcarrig House, Gorey, Co. Wexford. Tel. 055-25116. It provides sheltered work and living for mentally handicapped adults.

Grangemockler Camphill Community, Temple Michael, Grange-Mockler, Carrick-on-Suir, Co. Tipperary. A forty acre village for adults with special needs.

Rudolf Steiner Schools

The Holywood Rudolf Steiner School, 34, Croft Road, Holywood, Co. Down. Tel. Belfast 428029. The longest established Steiner School in Ireland, with both a Lower and an Upper School (Primary and Secondary), open to children from 4 to 18 years.

The Dublin Rudolf Steiner School, 28, Maxwell Road, Rathmines, Dublin 6. Tel. 01-960525. Begun in 1988, the Dublin School has a Kindergarten and Classes One, Two and Three, is open at present to children between the ages of 4 and 10 years and is expanding.

The Clare Rudolf Steiner School, Feakle, Co. Clare. Tel. 0619-21494. The Clare School is growing and at present is open to children between the ages of 4 and 12 years.

Biodynamic Farms

Information is available from: Anthony Kaye, Inisglas Trust, Crossabeg, Co. Wexford. Tel. 053-28226.

Practitioners of Anthroposophy

Down:

Dr. James Shank, 28, Princes Park, Holywood, Co. Down. BT18OPP. Tel. Holywood 5140. Anthroposophical Medicine and Eurythmy.

Cork:

Dr. Martin Lane, Millbrook Clinic, Bandon, Co. Cork. Tel. 023-41132. Family Doctor, Homoeopathy, Anthroposophical Medicine.

Tipperary:
Christine Maxwell, Dulcamara, Mullinahone, Co. Tipperary. Tel. 052-53256.
B.Sc., Medical Herbalist, Homoeopathic and Anthroposophical Medicine.

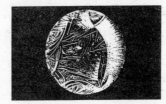

Chapter Ten

PSYCHOLOGICAL THERAPIES

Counselling Services in Ireland

by Eleanor O'Leary

There are many and diverse forms of Counselling, so many that it would require another book to clearly outline each method. The following article, "Counselling Services in Ireland" was written and compiled by Eleanor O'Leary, Ph.D., Director of the Guidance and Counselling Unit at the Department of Applied Psychology in University College, Cork. It has been previously published in the Institute of Guidance Counsellors Journal *of Autumn 1989.*

The range of professional and voluntary counselling services available in Ireland is a direct reflection of the incidence of various forms of social problems. People with problems of drug addiction, alcoholism, family/marital and sexual problems can profit from skilled counselling. Generally speaking, however, most socio-personal problems lend themselves to effective treatment by members of the counselling profession. Voluntary counselling services provide information and advice in addition to a supporting environment. Patterson (1971) states that the professional counsellor is someone who is skilled in working with clients with a preparation beyond that which the non-professional voluntary counsellor possesses. There is, however, very little agreement within psychology concerning the kind of training that justifies a person calling himself/herself a counsellor or psychotherapist. This was pointed out by the Professional Affairs of the British Psychological Society in 1981 and 1982.

The following are some of the types of counselling services available in Ireland at the present time:
1. **Guidance Counselling**
2. **Health Boards**

3. **Counselling Centres**
4. **Alcoholism and Drug Addiction Centres**
5. **Marriage and Family Therapy Centres**
6. **Voluntary Counselling Services**
7. **Counselling Psychologists in private practice**

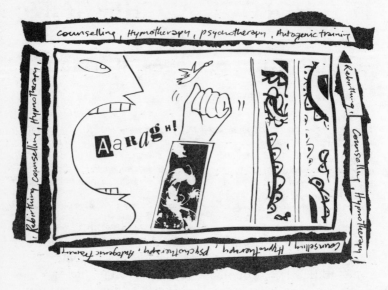

Guidance Counselling

In September 1989, there were 539 registered members of the Institute of Guidance Counsellors. These work in second level schools throughout the country and are engaged in individual and group counselling. Guidance counselling is the only professional counselling service which is organised at national level in Ireland. The therapies which are employed are mostly person-centred, for example *Gestalt and Heron's Six-Category Intervention Analysis, Psychosynthesis and Reality Therapy*. A study by O'Leary (1984) found that the problems dealt with by the guidance counsellor can be categorised as follows: (1) parent-child interaction; (2) adolescent reactions; (3) school environment; (4) personality problems. Guidance counsellors receive training for one year on a full-time basis. The course content includes counselling skills for both individual and group work.

Health Boards

The following is a geographical profile of the psychological services provided by the health boards in the Republic (Summer 1989).

AREA	NO OF CLINICAL PSYCHOLOGISTS	OTHER SERVICES
Eastern	1 Director of Psychology 4 Senior Clinical Psychologists 14 Basic Clinical Psychologists	1 Community Non-Clinical Psychologist
North-East	1 Senior Clinical Psychologist 2 Basic Clinical Psychologists	1 Community Non-Clinical Psychologist
South-East	1 Senior Clinical Psychologist 3 Basic Clinical Psychologists	Alcoholic Day Centre, St. Finbarr's Hospital, Cork (3 Counsellors)
Southern	2 Senior Clinical Psychologists 5 Basic Clinical Psychologists	3 Community Non-Clinical Psychologists
Western	1 Principal Psychologist 2 Senior Clinical Psychologists 8 Basic Clinical Psychologists	
Mid-Western	2 Senior Clinical Psychologists 3 Basic Clinical Psychologists	
North-West	1 Senior Clinical Psychologist 5 Basic Clinical Psychologists	
Midlands	2 Senior Clinical Psychologists 2 Basic Clinical Psychologists	St. Lomans Hospital (8 Counsellors)

Counselling Centres

Adam and Eve Counselling and Consultation Centre

4, Merchant's Quay, Dublin 8. Tel. 01-711910. This centre provides a personal, marital, family and vocational counselling service. A consultation and advisory service for relatives or friends of clients is also available. Problems dealt with range from neuroses to depression to schizoid personality disorders, from sexual-identity to post-abortion syndrome, from alcoholism to anxiety states. Therapies available include Psychoanalysis, Behaviour Modification, Gestalt Therapy and Logo-Therapy.

Guidance and Counselling Unit
Dept. of Applied Psychology, University College, Cork. Tel. 021-276871 ext. 2612. The Unit provides Professional Guidance, Counselling and Therapy for personal problems, communications problems, depression, anxiety. Gestalt Therapy, Transactional Analysis, Client-Centred Therapy and Sic-Category Intervention.

Mater Dei Youth Counselling Centre
Clonliffe Road, Dublin 3. Tel. 01-371892. The centre provides a vocational guidance and counselling service for young people at individual and group levels. Youth problems relating to physical and mental health, personal relationships, sexual identity, career choice, family relationships, school progress. Family Therapy, Group Therapy, Individual Counselling, Psychiatric Consultation and Therapy.

Creative Counselling Centre
7, Park Drive, Dun Laoghaire, Co. Dublin. Tel. 01-801671. Family Therapy, Marital Therapy, Individual Therapy, Gestalt Therapy, Deep Tissue Massage and neo-Reichian approaches.

Centre for Education Counselling and Psychotherapy
5, Fr. Mathew St., Cork. Tel. 021-274951. A professional counselling and psychotherapy service to individuals, couples, families and groups. Marital problems, loneliness, bereavement, depression, crises, pressure at work, unemployment, eating disorders, dependence on tranquillisers. Client-Centred, Psychodrama, Gestalt, Behaviour Modification and Family Therapy.

Dublin Well Woman Centre Ltd
73, Lr. Leeson St., Dublin 2. Tel. 01-789511; 60, Eccles St., Dublin 1. Tel. 01-728051. The centres provide professional counselling and advice for women on matters relating to

sexual health. Problems relating to the physical and mental aspects of sexual health. Various forms of therapy are used.

Eckhart House (Institute of Psychosynthesis)
19, Clyde Road, Dublin 4. Tel. 01-684687. Individual sessions are available for individuals experiencing existential crisis or deep-seated personality break-down. Crisis related to meaning in life, work project or vocation, inappropriate behaviour patterns. Psychosynthesis.

Dundalk Centre for Counselling/Personal Development
"Oakdene", Kincora Tce., Carrick Road, Dundalk, Co. Louth. Tel. 042-38333. The centre offers individual and group counselling, career assessment and guidance. Anxiety, depression, loneliness, relationship problems, alcohol. Individual Pastoral, Vocational and Therapeutic Counselling, Group Counselling.

Alcoholism and Drug Addiction Centres

Alcoholic Rehabilitation Centre
Golden Bridge House, Tyrconnell St., Dublin 8. Tel. 01-543793. The centre provides a specialised counselling service for alcoholics and an advisory service for relatives and friends. Alcoholism and the problems of rehabilitating alcoholics. Various therapies are employed.

Coolemine Lodge Therapeutic Centre
Coolemine, Clonsilla, Co. Dublin. Tel. 01-214545/216564. The centre provides a professional counselling service for alcoholics and drug addicts. Drug and alcohol addiction. Directive Therapy, Behaviour Modification, Positive Assertiveness Training.

Rutland Centre Ltd
Knocklyon House, Knocklyon Rd., Dublin 16. Tel. 01-946358. The centre provides a professional counselling service for alcoholics and drug addicts. Aftercare extends for a period of two years. Alcoholism and drug addiction. Group and Individual Therapy, Family/Marital Therapy.

Shelter Referral
The Merrion Centre, 288, Merrion Road, Dublin 4. Tel. 01-696033. The centre provides a professional counselling service and rehabilitation programme. Alcoholism. Individual/Family/Marital Counselling, Group Therapy, Social Skills Training.

Cuan Mhuire
Cordington, Athy, Co. Kildare. Tel. 0507-31564. Individual and group counselling. Alcoholism. Group Therapy, Work Therapy, Client-Centred Therapy, Alcoholism Crisis Counselling.

The Hanly Centre
Eblana Avenue, Dun Laoghaire, Co. Dublin. Tel. 01-809795. Crisis counselling for alcoholics and their families. Out reach programmes for schools, parents and community groups. Alcoholism. Alcoholism Crisis Counselling.

Alcoholism Service
O'Connell St., Ennis, Co. Clare. Tel. 065-28178. The service provides treatment for alcoholics and their families. The programme is run twice yearly beginning in January and September. Alcoholism and related family problems. Family Therapy, Group Therapy.

Alcoholism Counselling Service
Bishopsgate St., Mullingar. Tel. 044-48298. Treatment for alcoholics and their families. Alcoholism. Various forms of therapy are employed.

Drug Advisory and Treatment Centre
Jervis St., Dublin 1. Tel. 01-723145. Drug addiction treatment and advice. Drug addiction. Various methods of therapy are employed.

Marriage and Family Therapy Centres

Marriage Counselling Service
24, Grafton St, Dublin 2. Tel. 01-720341. The service provides a professional guidance centre and counselling centre as well

as a marital sexual dysfunction clinic. Problems in Marriage, Marital Therapy, Psychosexual counselling.

Marriage and Family Institute
5, Clare St., Dublin 2. Tel. 01-765371. Professional counselling and therapy for couples, individuals and families. Child Behaviour Problems, Marriage Difficulties, Sexual Problems, Adolescent Problems, Depression. Anxieties and Phobias, Addictions. Marital and Family Therapy, Psychosexual Therapy.

Voluntary Counselling Services

Catholic Marriage Advisory Council
55 Centres Nation-Wide
"Sunville", Kilrush Rd., Ennis, Co. Clare. Tel. 065-29777.
32, Harcourt St., Dublin 2. Tel. 01-780866.
34, Paul St., Cork. Tel. 021-275678.
Marriage counselling, pre-marriage education in relation-ships, natural family planning, fertility awareness service, marital breakdown, sexual problems, family planning.

The Samaritans
112, Marlborough St., Dublin 1. Tel. 01-727700.
Coach St., Cork. Tel. 021-271323.
"Sunville", Kilrush Rd., Ennis, Co. Clare. Tel. 065-29777.
2, St. Brendan's Ave., Wood Quay, Galway. Tel. 061-61222.
26, Upper Cecil St., Limerick. Tel. 061-42111.
13, Beau St., Waterford. Tel. 051-72114.
Listening Service. Suicide, loneliness, depression, marital problems, sexual abuse.

Rape Crisis Centres
70, Lr. Leeson St., Dublin 2. Tel. 01-614911.
27, McCurtain St., Cork. Tel. 021-968086.
P.O.Box 128, Limerick. Tel. 061-311511.
Support system for victims of rape or sexual assault. Counselling service. Sexual assault or rape, sexual harass-ment, child molestation.

Parents under Stress
Centre Care, Cathedral St., Dublin 1. Tel. 01-788344.
Feelings of aggression in parents towards their children.

Retirement Planning Council of Ireland
3, Lr. Leeson St., Dublin 2. Tel. 01-783600.
Problems in retirement. Financial problems.

Family Aid
P.O.Box 791, Dublin 1. Tel. 01-540055
Violence in the home.

Counselling Psychologists in private practice

There are a growing number of counsellors/psychologists in private practice throughout the country. Their techniques and perspectives, training and qualifications vary considerably. Details can generally be found in the local newspapers, telephone directories. The information in this article is intended to serve as a guide and the list provided is by no means complete. No evaluation of qualification or expertise in the area is intended.

References:
Client 'Drop-Out' in counselling. O'Leary E. (Institute of Guidance Counsellors Journal). 9. 16-19 1984.
Theories of Counselling and Psychotherapy. Patterson, C.M. (New York: Harper and Row). 1971.
Note: Re. Psychological Therapies, see also Tony Quinn Centres p. 216.

The Irish Association for Counselling

The Irish Association for Counselling (IAC) was established in 1981. The functions of the Association include the following: to represent counsellors in Ireland at national and international level; to provide a support and information system for counsellors and anyone interested in counselling; to set and maintain standards of training and practice; to provide a system of accreditation for counsellors.

Services to the Public

The IAC maintains a list of approved and accredited counsellors which is available to the general public. Counsellors on this list have undergone a rigorous vetting process which inquired into their training; experience; their commitment to personal development and their arrangements for supervision.

Accredited counsellors are required to have adequate arrangements for ongoing supervision and to subscribe to the IAC code of ethics and practice. In the event of a possible breach of this code of ethics and practice by an accredited counsellor, an aggrieved client is entitled to make representation to the secretary of the IAC.

The IAC office may be contacted at 01-801605. The Executive Committee of the IAC may be contacted at: 01-804424 (24 hours) 01-801671 (24 hours).

Grow Ireland

Grow is an international self and mutual help organisation. It operates mainly on a voluntary basis, with groups in most towns in Ireland. In Grow groups, people meet regularly to work through problems of any nature. The Grow Programme gives the philosophy of Grow as well as practical steps to be taken in order to grow out of difficult situations. Grow members are drawn from all walks of life and there are groups in some psychiatric hospitals. For further information contact: Grow Ireland, 11, Liberty St., Cork. Tel. 021-277520 or Grow Ireland, 50, Middle Abbey St., Dublin 1. Tel. 01-734029.

Northern Ireland Centres

Beginning Experience

Contact Bridie Gallagher, 4, Orphen Park, Kilfennen, Derry. Tel. Derry 47967. A self help group for separated, divorced and widowed which deals with specific problems as people work through the grief process and offers support and direction for the future.

Contact Youth Counselling Service

2a, Ribble St., Newtonards Rd., Belfast BT4 1HW. Tel. Phyllis Twamley, Belfast 57848. Drop-in and telephone Counselling

Service. A free confidential counselling service for young people who need someone impartial to talk to about the difficult areas in their lives. We encourage those coming to us to work towards a better understanding of themselves and their problems.

Lifespring
111, Cliftonville Rd., Belfast BT14. Tel. Belfast 753658. Psychotherapeutic counselling, specialising in working with the individual person in the context of their family of origin; resolution of intimate relationships; dependency issues; work with adult children of alcoholics; holistic approach to healing of mind, body, spirit and emotions. Work with terminally ill people and their families.

Life Cycle Centre
Dr. Stan Papenfus, 6, Knocknashima Rd., Downpatrick, BT30 6LB. Tel. Downpatrick 2372. Constructive Alternativism. Confidence training and inner development. Life Cycle books and tapes on anxiety, depression and other topics.

Northlands Centre
68, Northland Rd., Derry BT48 0AL. Tel. Derry 363011. Treatment, Education and research of alcohol and other drugs. Advice, assessment, counselling and residential treatment.

Rape Crisis Centre
P.O.Box 46, Belfast BT2 7AR Tel. Belfast 249696.

Women's Aid
Regional Office, 143a University St., Belfast BT7 1HP. Tel. Belfast 249041.

Coleraine Womens Aid
3&3a, Abbey St., Coleraine, BT52 1DF.

Hypnotherapy

by Dr. Anjum Madani, M.B., B.Ch., B.A.O.,L.R.C.P.S.I.

Anjum Madani *is a General Practitioner whose main area of practise is Hypnotherapy and Psychotherapy. He lives and works in Dublin and is a member of the Irish Council for Hypnotic Psychotherapy and Counselling.*

Hypnotherapy is the utilisation of the hypnotic trance state by specific techniques to produce therapeutic change. It is imperative that we examine hypnosis in this context and liberate it from the shackles of myth, fear and prejudice. Trance states, being as they are a natural human experience, have been effectively used for healing purposes since time immemorial. All races and cultures have hypnotherapists but we shall restrict ourselves to an account of Modern Western Hypnosis.

It was in 1736 that Franz Anton Mesmer, an Austrian, having recently graduated in Medicine began to apply in his clinical practise the theories of *Animal Magnetism*. He affected astounding results with illnesses hitherto considered incurable by the medical profession of the time and his reputation spread all over Europe. Such was his impact that King Louis XVI appointed a Royal Commission to investigate *Mesmerism* in 1784. Among its members were Lavoisier, the famous chemist and Benjamin Franklin, the American statesman and scientist.

Predictably, no physical scientific basis for Mesmer's claims were discovered and his results were explained away as being brought about by imagination and imitation on the part of the patients. Mesmerism fell into disrepute and the medical profession adopted a hard uncompromising stand discouraging official advances in the field.

Notwithstanding this, physicians, surgeons, lay hypnotists, dentists, neurologists and psychiatrists contrived to use the techniques obtaining in most cases vast benefits and, in some, spectacular results. Unable to stem the tide of ever increasing numbers of respected professionals endorsing the, by now, well developed practise of hypnotherapy, the British Medical Association had no option but to appoint a new Commission to investigate the discipline. In 1953 the subcommittee published its report recommending that hypnosis be taught to physicians, psychiatrists, anaesthetists and obstetricians throughout England.

The British Society for Medical and Dental Hypnosis was formed in 1955 — the first of its kind. Today there are over thirty National Societies of Hypnosis world-wide with a rapidly growing body of knowledge about the hypnotic state and its utilisation for therapy and healing.

The essence of Hypnosis is the experience of a mental state of powerfully focused inner concentration and altered perception, combined with deep physical relaxation. There is no question of mind control or surrendering one's will to the therapist. Nor can the client be coerced to engage in acts against their will despite the dramatic performances of Stage Hypnotists, who, incidentally, have contributed to the misrepresentation of the discipline. The client retains both consciousness and the capacity to terminate the trance at will if so desired. Hypnosis is in fact a skill, not of the therapist, but of the client. The therapist is a trainer, a facilitator, not a manipulator as was so often wrongfully portrayed by the media in the past.

The potential for therapy lies in the ease with which access to the unconscious mind is gained. With the advancement of science and increasing understanding of the material world, humankind has attained greater control over the environment than primitive man could ever have imagined. But the mind has remained stoically defiant in yielding to man's probing search for Knowledge.

Even today, neuropsychological research reveals that while engaged in a task requiring total maximum concentration, only 10% of the brain appears to be activated; 90% remains dormant. We tend to call this the unconscious, that vast submerged part of our mind not immediately available to scrutiny.

Psychological problems initially manifest themselves in the conscious part of our mind from which they rapidly filter into the consciousness. At times, the conscious may be entirely bypassed, the problem embedding itself directly into the unconscious defying all attempts at removal. This, simplified, is how habits are formed — not just smoking or other addictive behaviour, but also erroneous pathways of thought, emotion and behaviour. Psychological problems automatically affect behaviour in some way. Thus, anxiety states, obsessive-compulsive disorders, phobias, hysterical conversions, depression etc. all manifest themselves physically.

Certain physical illnesses in their turn are susceptible to psychological states — the psychosomatic illnesses. Hence, asthma, angina, hypertension, irritable bowel syndrome, peptic ulcer, etc., if not brought on, are most certainly aggravated by emotion and stress. To complicate the scenario further, certain diseases can alter healthy mental states. The person suffering from chronic pain, or a cancer, though initially not depressed, will soon succumb to the inevitable toll on the psyche. This is the somato-psychic state, one not talked of frequently but of equal importance as the psychosomatic illnesses.

Under hypnosis, the conscious and the unconscious mind can be steadily trained to modify its influence on pathological processes be they physical or psychic. The result is greater control over physical symptoms and eradication of the vicious circle of incorrect thought — emotion — behaviour pathways that cause distress. In the hands of appropriately and ethically trained therapists, hypnosis can be a potent tool for facilitating a holistic healing process.

Psychotherapy

by Dr. Bernard Stein,M.B., M. Med Sc.(Psychotherapy), MISCE(Hypnosis)

Bernard Stein *is a Psychotherapist and Hypnotherapist. He lives and works in Dublin and is a member of the Irish Council for Hypnotic Psychotherapy and Counselling.*

Many people, at some time, experience a crisis or an ongoing problem in their encounter with the world, with other people, or within themselves. These conflicts may be manifested in the form of painful emotional or bodily feelings, and even physical illness. They may lead to strange subjective feelings.

One may experience a frightening feeling of unreality, as well as a loss (or lack) of a sense of self, of identity, of one's boundaries, of one's rights, or perhaps one may only be aware of a general sense of failure, resentment, fear, guilt, and poor self-esteem and loss of control.

In an effort to overcome these difficulties, many unsuccessfully resort to tablets, drugs or alcohol, and trade dependency and addiction for a partial alleviation of their problem which often re-appears. Old patterns continue unchanged 'dulled' but leading to a perpetuation of a pathogenic (that engenders illness) internal or external mental environment.

Many different models have been invented in an attempt to describe and make sense of the wide range of mental, emotional, behavioural and relational patterns and disorders that arise. These models provide a framework, within which 'malfunction' can be described and defined, and they suggest ways of correcting these 'malfunctions'.

None of these models contains *the truth*, i.e. the only right way of describing what is happening, (though some would claim to), but many of them provide a useful framework for change and relief from distress. Just as there are many ways to paint, or describe a picture, so there are many ways to describe how the mind works. Each model defines a different school, often named after the person who proposed it, (such as *Freudian, Jungian, Rogerian, Groffian*, etc.) or after a central aspect of the theory, (such as *Behavioural, Constructivist, Family, Gestalt, Rebirthing, Cognitive*, and so forth). It would be beyond the range of this introduction to describe them all, or to expand on any one of them.

There are descriptive terms which link several psychotherapies loosely together. Some are cognitive in that they encourage a deeper insight or understanding of the problem. They may be analytical, and intrapsychic in that they may go looking into the patient's past to find, through the unconscious, the seeds of the present dysfunction (e.g. psychoanalysis, hypnoanalysis, etc.), or they may be experiential, helping one to relive old traumas, and make new sense out of them, allowing a working through and a healing resolution to occur. Or, they may be systemic therapies, that disregard the past. These describe the problem as a manifestation of the system of interactions which the client participates in with other significant people, in the present. The roles the client enacts are central, in systemic therapy.

Some therapies, such as client centred or Rogerian therapy, emphasise the qualities the therapist must display, (such as empathy, positive regard, etc). At the other extreme, some therapies, are very prescriptive, such as some systemic approaches, behavioural approaches, some forms of hypnosis, and other forms of therapy that prescribe tasks. They vary as to whether they emphasise the need for insight and understanding to be gained from doing the task.

Some therapists seek change without insight. Many consider this type of therapy as *manipulative*, but proponents would emphasise that the rapid results justify the means. There is a risk of the therapist being cast in the role of a performer of miracles, which might have certain effects on the therapist's 'ego', and on the client's ability to take responsibility for him/herself.

Therapies also vary in whether they are practised on a one to one basis, or in groups, longterm or shortterm, whether they are problem centred, or whether they have the broad aim of developing one's human potential and personality.

Together with an experienced therapist, clients can often extricate themselves from the painful corner they feel trapped in. Through non-manipulative therapies, they can overcome self deceptions, forgive old hurts, forgive themselves, re-examine their dependencies and their assumptions about life, define their boundaries, and acknowledge their true feelings. They can escape old patterns of behaviour and interaction that were limiting and hurtful to them. They may thus explore new life strategies in a safe context, and let go of symptoms. They will then enjoy a new sense of themselves, of freedom to live and to be truthful and responsible for their lives. They will also experience an intuitive knowledge of what used to baffle them.

The author recommends that you choose a therapist who has undergone therapy, or has extensive experience of meaningful change in his/her own life. Such a person will have been through what he/she expects you to go through, and will be a more effective facilitator of change as a result.

It is important that you are aware of the credentials of anyone calling themselves a psychotherapist. There are no guarantees, but qualifications do provide some reassurance. The wrong choice can be costly, and potentially dangerous. In Ireland there are at present no regulations to prevent anyone from setting up and practising as a psychotherapist. A controversy over the difference between counselling and psychotherapy — there is quite a grey area between the two — exists. Counselling can be carried out quite effectively by people who have been trained for a relatively short period of time. It involves mainly good listening skills, and an ability to reflect back a person's ideas, as opposed to psychotherapy which normally involves a prolonged course of study and training, and follows a more clearly and elaborately defined philosophical structure. To elaborate on the many kinds of counsellors and therapists, and on the varying degrees of training and different approaches involved, would require another book!

Finally, not all problems described above require the help of a psychotherapist. Many problems can be helped or even resolved, by simply talking to a good neighbour whom you trust, a friend or your family doctor. Sadly, it is often difficult to find someone who can listen the way you need to be heard.

Practitioners

The Council for Hypnotic Psychotherapy and Counselling (CHPC) was formed in 1989 to:

— provide qualified ethical hypnotic psychotherapists with a Council
— maintain and make a national register of accredited members available to the public.
— promote awareness of hypnotic psychotherapy as a discipline for bringing about psychological change and for relieving varied psychological problems
— co-operate with other psychotherapeutic disciplines for the advancement of psychotherapy in general.

The CHPC sets and fosters high professional standards of hypnotic psychotherapy and allied disciplines by promoting seminars, workshops, and other forms of teaching in Ireland.

A future aim of the Council is to provide a syllabus of training in these subjects.

The CHPC has an established code of ethics which all members accept as binding. Members who are engaged in hypnotic psychotherapy and allied disciplines are pledged to provide treatment in the best therapeutic interests of the client, to respect the confidentiality of the client, and to protect the trust which the client invests in the member. Information regarding members of the CHPC in any particular area may be requested by contacting: Secretary, James Ronan, 30, Cherry Ave., Rathingle, Swords, Co. Dublin. Tel.404161.

CHPC Members

Dublin:
Josie Hogarty, "High Breeze", Ballyedmonduff, Sandyford, Co. Dublin. Tel. 01-954251; also 4, Waldemar Tce., Dundrum.
Type of work: Hypnotic Psychotherapy (Clinical one to one.)
Analytic Psychotherapy (Group).
Qualifications: C.H. (Cert of Hypnosis),D.H.P. (Diploma of Hypnotherapy and Psychotherapy).
Frank Mc Ardle, 22, Rathgar Ave., Rathgar, Dublin 6. Tel. 986589.
Type of work: Counselling/Deep Relaxation. Alcoholism, Emotional, Personal, Relationships, A.C.O.A.(Adult Children Of Alcoholics).
Qualifications: Certificate Substance Abuse/Addiction Studies, Certificate Personal Skills, Diploma in Counselling, Certificate Alcoholism Counselling (Chicago 1978).
Dr. Anjum Madani, 106, South Circular Road, Dublin 8. Tel. 532816.
Type of work: Hypnotherapy and Psychotherapy.
Qualifications: M.B.B.Cl., B.A.O., L.R.C.P.&S.I. General Practitioner.
Aidan Maloney, 76, Pine Valley Ave., Rathfarnham, Dublin 16. Tel. 01-946009.
Type of work: Psychotherapy, Management Consultant, Neuro-Linguistic-Programming.
Qualifications: M.A., Dip. Stats.
Alan Mooney, 42, Strand St., Skerries, Co. Dublin. Tel. 01-491209.
Type of work: Psychotherapy — Gestalt, bio-energetics, non-directive hypnotherapy. Does not work with addiction to drugs, drink or food. Will refer clients to other agencies.
Qualifications: M.I.C. (Scotland).
James Ronan, 30, Cherry Ave., Rathingle, Swords, Co. Dublin. Tel. 01-404161.
Type of work: Hypnotherapy.
Qualifications: Four years theory, practice, workshops, specialist reading.
Dr. Bernard Stein, Belgrave Psychotherapy Centre, 1, Charleston Rd., Rathmines, Dublin 6. Tel. 01-975666.
Type of work: Counsellor, Psychotherapist, Hypnotherapist.
Qualifications: M.B., M.Med. Sc.(Psychotherapy), MISCE (Hypnosis).
Dr. Joseph Robinson, Polehore, Killurin, Wexford. Tel. 053-28181.
Type of work: Hypnotherapy and Psychotherapy.
Qualifications: Ph.D., F.I.M.L.S.

Independent Practitioners

Centres

The Family Therapy and Counselling Centre

55, Ranelagh Village, Dublin 6. Tel. 01-971188. Hours 9.00 to 5.30. Monday to Friday, evenings and Saturday by appointment; This is a group practice of Family Therapy and Counselling for individuals; eating disorders, personal development, relationships, depression, habit control, phobias. Couples; marital conflict, communication difficulties, sexual problems, mediation service for separating couples. Families; difficulties with adolescents, school related and family problems. Members of the practise are Registered Family Therapists with additional qualifications in Law, Occupational Therapy and Social Work. The fees charged vary according to the income of the client/s.

The Vico Consultation Centre

6, Charlemont Tce., Crofton Road, Dun Laoghaire, Dublin. Tel. 01-843336; The Vico Consultation Centre is a Mental Health Care Organisation providing consultation and training services as follows: psychotherapeutic, psychological and psychiatric services which include assessments, consultations and therapy for children, adults, couples, families and groups; training, supervision and consultation with professionals in health and social services; consultation with professional, health care and business organisations, as well as with social service agencies and schools. Training workshops in Systemic-Constructivist therapy. Consultations are available in French, Dutch or German, as well as in English. Fees are open to negotiation.

The Pet Bereavement Advisory Service

Aine Wellard, 7b Moss St., Dublin 2. Tel. 01-775097. Aine Wellard is a psychologist with additional training in counselling and psychosynthesis. The Advisory Service offers a specialised counselling service for pet bereavement for adults and children. Sessions last from one hour to 90 minutes and the fee is £15.

Southern Ireland Practitioners

Cork:
J.Keaney, Cork Hypnotherapy Clinic, Tuckey House, 8,Tuckey St., Cork. Tel. 021-273575; Suggestion Therapy (for smoking, slimming, nailbiting, etc.), Relaxation, help with fears, phobias, and anxiety, Analytical Therapy.

Northern Ireland Practitioners

Belfast:
Alan Gilchrist, Belfast Hypnotherapy Centre, 409, Lisburn Rd., Belfast BT97EW; also 4 Wellington St., Ballymena BT43 6AD; Tel. Belfast 667982 (business hours) 301204 (evenings).
Liz Comerton, 28, Hampton Park, Belfast, BT4 3JN Tel. 643630.
Type of work: Reike, Relaxation, Yoga, Look Good — Feel Good, Building Self-Confidence, Stress Management; Duration of Session: One hour and a half; Fee : £15 individual.
Donegal:
Jane Mountain, Meitheal Centre, Inch Island, Co. Donegal, Tel. 077-60323; *Type of work:* Assertiveness Training, Relaxation, Woman-oriented counselling and therapy; Qualifications : B.Sc.(Social Science), C.Q.S.W.
Paul Swann, Meitheal Centre, Inch Island, Co. Donegal, Tel. 077-60323; also at 21, Bishop St., Derry, Tel. Derry 266610.
Type of work: Creative Meditation and Visualisation Practices for relaxation, concentration, self-confidence, improved relationships, creative lifestyle, personal growth.
(see Meitheal Centre, p. 209)

Autogenic Training

Autogenic Training is a series of mental exercises designed to switch off the 'fight or flight' system of the body, and switch on the rest and relaxation system. It was developed in Germany by Dr. Johannes Schultz in the 1930s and is now widely used as a way of combating stress.

In autogenics, the mind is trained to influence the body, applying principles similar to those of Yoga, self-hypnosis and auto-suggestion. By focusing on different parts and functions of the body, such as the limbs, circulation, breathing, a deep state of physical and mental calm is achieved. The exercises can be self-taught but are generally learned during a programme of weekly sessions. Sessions last from one to one and a half hours, and exercises are carried out three times daily during training. They involve visualisation as well as physical and mental relaxation. There are generally applicable exercises as well as exercises that can be developed to help with specific complaints.

Once mastered, the exercises can be practised virtually anywhere, at any time — in bed, in the bath, sitting up or lying down. In effect, Autogenic Training teaches how to achieve a deep state of relaxation. It is widely understood that stress is a physical as well as an emotional reality, and that relaxation not only helps to prevent stress, but works in a positive way for mind and body.

People who suffer from stress related and psychosomatic problems including the following have been shown to benefit from Autogenic Training: anxiety and tension, asthma, depression, drug dependency, insomnia, menopausal difficulties, pre-menstrual tension, problems with smoking or drinking. Autogenics, by helping us to relax, also permits us to be more creative and alert, and to cope better with the demands of daily life.

Practitioners

Edward Boyne, Tel. 01-809178 (24 hours) 01-801671 (24 hours).
Dr. Brian Kennedy, Tel. 01-683996, also Homoeopathy.
Turning Point, Tel. 01-680588.
Joan Tyndall, Tel. 01-956126.

Autogenic Training Classes
Autogenic Training classes are held regularly in Dublin City Centre and Dun Laoghaire. For further details, telephone 01-809178, 01-801671 (24 hours).

Chapter Eleven

REBIRTHING

by Richard Waterborn

Richard Waterborn *is a Re-Birther and member of the Association of Irish Re-Birthers who lives and works in Cork.*

Rebirthing is a safe, powerful tool for personal growth, healing and transformation, based on a technique called Conscious Connected Breathing. Whilst its roots can be traced back to the ancient esoteric Yogic traditions of the East, rebirthing in its present form was rediscovered in the early 1970s and has been widely taught and practised in the West since 1976. The aim is to gently let go of physical, mental and emotional blocks in our life, arising from birth and early experience, resulting in a joyful integration of energies and an enhanced capacity to live life fully and freely.

Birth is our introduction to the world, and for all of us involves a certain amount of trauma as we leave behind the warm, secure and supportive reality of the womb and move, often painfully into a radically different environment, full of strange and intense stimuli. In the midst of this momentous transition we are required to take our first breath and not surprisingly, this is usually an agonised gasp, forced upon us by direct necessity, rather than a voluntary, pleasurable act.

Recent scientific and medical findings have demonstrated that the pre and peri-natal infant is a highly sensitive and aware being, biologically designed for extremely rapid and deep learning. Events from birth and early infancy exert a strong conditioning influence upon us, leading to lasting decisions as to the nature of reality. These often negative experiences are reinforced by interaction with our parents and other key figures in the world and become the foundation of our personal belief systems. Fear, pain, struggle, separation from the source of love and security, are just some of the emotions associated with our first impressions of the world. Since these emotions arouse such intense, life threatening anxiety, they are rapidly suppressed into the unconscious, only to resurface later in our lives as inexplicable feelings of anxiety, guilt, anger, alienation and frustration, as the source of conflict and difficulty in relationships or as the root of phobias, neuroses and psychoses.

Conscious Connected Breathing when practised in the presence of a trained rebirther, frees the full breathing mechanism trapped since birth, energises the whole body system, and initiates a profound biological healing process. Accumulated tensions and fears from early life are brought to our conscious awareness and gently dissolved by the breathing rhythm. Experiences originally thought to be too life threatening and hence suppressed are safely and easily integrated into consciousness, bringing a deep sense of release, well-being and peace.

As we let go of these resistances to the totality of our lives, we experience the bliss of pure existence, and the vital energy previously locked up in suppression is regained for our increased enjoyment of life. On the mental level, we become aware of habitual unconscious beliefs and complexes which create highly charged negative emotions and keep us locked into disease, guilt, suffering and misery. Having released deeply embedded negative attitudes, we are free to make conscious choices about present life experiences which were previously dealt with compulsively, since the accumulated tensions limited our choice. We become free and powerful creators of our own lives. Moving backwards through the core events of our past we may re-experience the actual circumstances of our birth, and the letting go of such birth-related tensions is so dramatically complete that the term re-birth has been chosen to describe it.

Some Questions about Rebirthing:

Is it a religion or cult?
Rebirthing has no religious or sectarian content, although it has been described as a biological experience of God! While

most people experience a deepening of their own particular spiritual focus, rebirthing supports each individual in learning to trust their internal judgement and intuition rather than becoming dependent on an external personality or organisation.

Do I have to re-enact my birth?

With the growing awareness that birth is the single most impacting event of our lives (recognised by Freud and most major psychologists since), a number of therapies have been developed which seek in some way to physically simulate the birth experience. Rebirthing does not rely on any such techniques, nor does it require a person to imagine, or attempt to re-enact their birth.

Will I have to keep doing it for years?

Rebirthing works fast! While it is recommended to do at least 10 sessions with a qualified rebirther, people are encouraged to become sufficiently familiar and safe with the process to practise it for themselves. However, since it is so pleasurable and beneficial, most people choose to continue rebirthing as a regular part of their lives.

Who is it suitable for?

Rebirthing is of benefit to absolutely everyone who wishes to change or improve the quality of their lives and relationships. It has also been extremely successful in healing specific physical and psychological disorders by identifying and releasing the mental/emotional condition underlying the manifest symptoms. Rebirthing is highly recommended for prospective parents, and is an invaluable preparation for childbirth.

What happens in a Rebirthing session?

A typical rebirthing session lasts between two and three hours, during which the client lies down and goes through a full connected breathing cycle, lasting anywhere between sixty and ninety minutes. The rest of the session is taken up with reviewing the client's progress and counselling, to maximise the benefit of the breathing cycle and, to complete, a mutual assessment and clarification of the client's experience.

How much does it cost?
The cost of a rebirthing session varies between £20-£40 depending largely on the rebirther's degree of experience and qualification. Many rebirthers are willing to negotiate their fee or trade services in order to facilitate people who want to be rebirthed.

How can I begin Rebirthing?
There is a growing number of professional rebirthers practising in Ireland. In addition, many rebirthers offer one-day seminars and weekend workshops on various topics associated with rebirthing, such as Birth or Relationships, and also organise workshops for seminar leaders and trainers from other countries.

Practitioners

AIR — The Association of Irish Rebirthers
AIR is an organisation and information centre which supports and promotes the Rebirthing Profession in Ireland. Membership is open to anyone working or intending to work as a professional Rebirther.

Full details of membership and registration requirements as well as information about forthcoming workshops and training are available from: Secretary, Patsy Brennan, Rear 4, Crofton Terrace, Dunlaoghaire, Dublin. Tel. 01-841660.

Members of AIR

Cork:
Richard Waterborn, Lios na Greine, 9, Sunmount, Military Hill, Cork. Tel. 021-505422; Eleanor O'Flynn. Tel. 021-372126.
Down:
Helen Johnston, 7a, Clifton Rd., Bangor, Co. Down. Tel. Bangor 453411.
Dublin:
Patsy Brennan, Rear 4, Crofton Terrace, Dun Laoghaire, Dublin. Tel. 01-841660; Brenda Doherty. Tel. 01-422460; also Aromatherapy; Kathleen Hogan. Tel. 01-881725; Oliver Tatten. Tel. 01-976553; Carol Walker, 11, Eskar Park, Lucan, Co. Dublin. Tel. 01-241810.
Wicklow:
Steve Gregory and Trish Cameron, Keenan's Cottage, Red Lane, Lower

Calary, Bray, Co. Wicklow. Tel 01-875330. Both are also Counsellors and Trish practises Women's Healing. Judith Crowe, The Heritage, Newtownmountkennedy, Co. Wicklow. Tel. 01-819515. Also teaches Birth Preparation for mothers and couples, pre-natal Yoga and will attend births to assist the midwife and parent/s.
England:
Binnie Dansby, 18, Cottesmore Gardens, Kensington, London W8.

List of Independent Practitioners
Donegal:
Peter Francis, Meitheal Centre, Inch Island, Donegal. Tel. 077-60323. Also Spiritual Healer.

List of Northern Ireland Practitioners

The Rebirth Centre, 50, Duncairn Gardens, Belfast BT15. Tel. Sara Reid, Belfast 748089.
Mary Grant, Lifespring, 111, Cliftonville Rd., Belfast BT14. Tel. Belfast 753658. Also teaches and practises Aromatherapy, practises Massage, Counselling and is the Co-ordinator of Lifespring; Sighia Mary O'Donoghue, Shambhala, 7, Ashley Gardens, Belfast BT15 4DU. Tel. Belfast 771104. Also Massage-Bodywork, Integration counselling and therapy.

Chapter Twelve

SPIRITUAL HEALING

Introduction

Faith Healing has a long tradition in Ireland and has been practised both inside and outside of the main religions here. In that tradition it is understood that faith itself is the healer — the faith of the healer, and his or her gift of healing. Sceptics have argued that it is the faith of the recipient that heals and that illnesses healed in this way tend to re-occur.

During the past ten years, however, Spiritual Healing has become more and more widely taught and availed of and is practised in different ways. The most common of these is based on the Oriental wisdom that each living thing has an aura, or energy field, around it, which can be felt with the hands, seen by some people and photographed by using Kirlian photography. The aura emanates from the physical body and the emotions, but also links our material life to the spiritual realm. The aura gives and receives energy, or vibrations, to and from all living things, as do the chakras.

There are seven chakras, in a line from the top of the head to the base of the spine. The word *chakra* means wheel in Sanskrit. The chakras are the dynamic centres of the different kinds of energies and of the senses. In photographs and drawings, the aura and chakras are extraordinarily beautiful, colourful and flowing. Spiritual Healing is sometimes practised in Ireland in a way that has become, to my mind, packaged, commercialised, and mystified. The deeper Spiritual Healing will engage the recipient in self under-standing and self-healing and will involve an awareness that illness has resulted from a denial of the higher self.

Some Spiritual Healers work from the understanding that the individual human spirit incarnates and re-incarnates in a physical body in order to evolve. It is said that the Earth is simultaneously both the most joyous and the most difficult

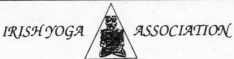

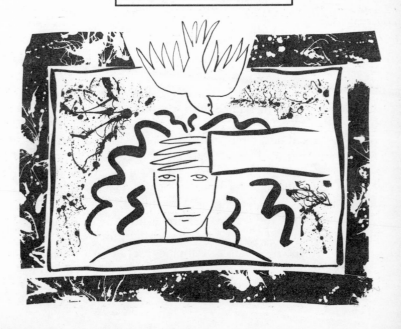

plane of existence. The concept of incarnation and re-incarnation is incomplete without the concept *Karma*. It is one's Karma to manifest and express one's special gifts, to take one's special place on this Earth and also to undo or neutralise any errors made during the spirit's evolution. The individual spirit undertakes such a journey not just for the sake of its own evolution, but because it is born of and returns to Universal Love and the purpose of Love, is to love.

Other traditions hold, not that there is continuity of the individual spirit in successive incarnations, but, that the spiritual realm manifests itself in different forms at different times and that it is a collective and universal evolution that has also been undertaken, in the name of Love.

Recently, a scientific interest in the energy fields has emerged and it has become possible to measure and influence the energy fields of living things by means of instrumentation as well as by using the hands. It would be ironic indeed if that work was to diminish the recognition of the importance of the consciousness and the will in our understanding and treatment of illness. Ironic because its foundations are in a tradition where awareness is the first and the last step to be taken for the full realisation of our potential as human and as spirit.

Finally, the remainder of this introduction is a sort of an explanation as to why a French practitioner has contributed to *Sláinte!*

I first met M. Levillain in August 1987. I was spending summer holidays in France with my family. Before going, I had written to a friend there, a practitioner and teacher of Shiatsu. I asked her to please find someone on the alternative medicine scene who could cure me of psoriasis. I had had psoriasis on and off since my mid-teens. I had used steroid creams, Ultra Violet A treatment, and even been hospitalised for two weeks during Dithranol treatment. The treatments were worse than the psoriasis in my estimation — although that was pretty bad. Physically, it was sore, and covered large areas of my body. I was developing psoriatic rheumatism, particularly noticeable during the winter months. I was living an active life by any standards, but I was unhappy in it. Restless, looking for answers and in particular wanting to know why I had psoriasis. It seemed that the medical explanation that my skin was growing in a different way from most people's didn't really answer that question: 'Psychosomatic'; 'hereditary'; 'adolescent trauma'; 'present or incipient in 10% of the population of the Northern Hemisphere', best of all 'psoriasis : as harmless as freckles'.

Louise drove me through acres of sunflowers to visit Louis-Guy, one August morning early. After introductions at his house, I lay face-down on a standard healer's couch. Louis-Guy passed his hands slowly over my body from head to toe, without touching, not missing any part. Gradually, everything, big or small, that I was worried or tense about came into my mind, and evaporated. I felt that I was being cleansed of a lifetime of guilt, misapprehension, self-doubt, fear, anger, loneliness. Instead peace, joy, love, forgiveness, acceptance and belonging were released.

I lay face down, looking to my left at an open window that let in a shaft of sunlight onto the marble floor, a French bird called, the window was framed with greenery and slowly, slowly, I began to fly. Up and up over the Pyrennees, and still upward, until only the sky was visible. I had closed my eyes, the better to see my flying companion and the celestial scenery. There was nothing but the heavens. Sure at last that I wasn't going to fall, or be punished, for my curiosity, I opened my eyes to see what had become of the room. It was still there, but I was also still flying. Much later, we came down slowly and were still. I had one more treatment from Louis-Guy that week, and came home to Ireland.

Gradually, my skin began to heal. I read about Spiritual Healing, in particular *Practising the Presence* and *The Art of Spiritual Healing* and other works by Joel Goldsmith, and began to practise meditation. I have had one bad relapse of psoriasis since then which Louis-Guy treated on a visit to Ireland. This healing made such a difference to my life on every level that I was prompted to further explore the whole area of healing. I had become resigned to living with psoriasis and the discovery that this was not necessary lead me to compiling this book, in the hope that others too will discover the possibility of healing, by whatever method or methods suit their circumstances and outlook on life.

Faith Healer

by Louis-Guy Levillain

Louis-Guy Levillain *lives in Mirepoix, in France. He is a Spiritual Healer, a Magnetist, a teacher of Aikido and works in conjunction with practitioners of other disciplines who live nearby. His account of how he became a Healer is translated from French. He says that these lines are written in the hope that they will help '. . . those who, one day, will work from a faith in love and abundance.'*

I was brought up by my father, a railway worker, and my grandparents. I was a teenager during the '60s and I was actively involved in the political revolution of 1968, in Communist and Trade Union organisations. In 1970 I turned away from that and moved to the south of France. There I met people whose lifestyle was completely different from what I had known before and who were looking for a society based on love. There I met my wife and in 1973 she gave birth to our first child, Jonathan. I was extremely happy; I was ready to change the world in order to offer it to this being who came from us.

When Jonathan was two years old he had a serious illness affecting the throat. The doctor called frequently but when Jonathan continued having fits we were at a loss as to what to do. We were living on a caravan site and all of the inhabitants, including myself, worked in the big shipyards on the Belgian border. One morning, our neighbour, a docker in Dunkirk, came to see us and proposed that we should pray for Jonathan to be healed. I accepted his suggestion although I did not believe in his healing ability. One evening he came with cakes and his bible. He opened his bible at random, put his right hand on my child's head and began to read a verse that lasted for 10 minutes. The following morning Jonathan was much better, and was cured 3 days later. Thus began for me the long journey in the understanding of the Divine. This man belonged to a religion, a religion that gave people access to healing. I couldn't get over it, I didn't believe in it but I developed a close interest in this church that had opened my eyes to a living God. For a year I attended prayer meetings every Sunday. I came to know the bible and the life of Jesus and I found the Adepts of this church awe-inspiring and full of Faith.

In 1976, we decided to move to another region where I found another prayer hall that belonged to the same group. However, one evening during the month of May, Jonathan had a high fever. The doctor had diagnosed meningitis and predicted that he would be dead in forty-eight hours. When I arrived at around eleven o'clock at night, Jonathan was lying stiff in the bed, his eyes were rolling and the mounting fever was making him delirious. I knelt down at the foot of his bed and raised my arms to heaven. I cried aloud to God to save my child. Five minutes later Jonathan sat up without any fever, as if nothing had happened.

This was the second instance where Grace came to open my eyes. My fervour and devotion to God led me to give up the job so far away. I began to work instead on a nearby farm which left me with much more free time. I returned early to the house, and attended prayer meetings throughout the week and spoke to all of my friends about how this love of God could change my life. Four months after this wonderful act, I decided to become a Pastor and to study. I asked a friend to advise me.

He proposed that I should fast for two days of prayer, reread the new testament and be baptised, which I did. After the baptism I attended the Monday evening prayer meetings which were reserved for the most fervent and it was at one of those meetings that I received the third Grace. Three Pastors read the bible aloud with their right hands on my head. I too began to speak aloud, even louder than they, without a Bible, in a language that I did not know. And I couldn't stop myself; someone else in the hall translated the message. Then a large light appeared a little way behind me, a transparent bluish light, an awesome light, with a figure inside it that I can only describe as sexless. At the same time, I received a Force of Love that no human being could give, an intense sweetness enveloped me, an inner joy that brought tears from my eyes, and I spoke all the time, and faster, without understanding. I don't know how long this lasted, all I remember is that I was transcended. Until August 1977 I shared and gave to others all that I had. At that time, we lived in a small presbytery and our second baby was due. At the beginning of August, the curate asked me to leave, because the villagers could not tolerate my competing with the church.

We agreed to go elsewhere so that this second child would be born in good circumstances. We found another place where I made new friends. They followed a different path from mine, which I had believed to be the only one of its kind; they studied Zen Buddhism. They taught me of Karma and Meditation; I taught them the Love of Christ and of how to know truth by the Presence of God. This did not please the head Pastor, who came to my house and demanded that I choose between the church to which I belonged and that of the others. I responded that nothing had changed, that God is in everybody, that it does not matter which is the principal church, it is only important that a man should be strong in his Faith in order to bring more Universal Love. Then I separated from the group in whose church I felt a prisoner.

My wife was not sympathetic to my spiritual life and for four years, living together was very hard. I had set myself up as a craftsman and started a building business. The knowledge of Zen lead me to practise the Martial Arts. So it went until 1987, switching from mystic to businessman, from smalltime craftsman to entrepreneur. In April 1987 my wife and I separated. I had started the Martial Arts without practising seriously. I felt that the time had come to dedicate my life to what I liked best: the search for my identity.

Through Aikido, I learned to transcend pride, egotism, passion, etc., to know the Force of Ki, of Hara in Yoga, and the Chakras. In 1984, I began to teach Aikido, and students also came for spiritual teachings, for explanations of their bodies and understanding of the Cosmic and Universal. They came too for a type of Magnetism that I passed to them (they said) and it was at that time that I began to treat injuries, sprains, sicknesses and any ailment you can think of. Some were relieved, others healed. The number of students increased and I felt myself to be more of a spiritual instructor than a corrector of movement. I sought more to liberate the spirit in self-acceptance and acceptance of others than to teach movement. I felt that I should make my students conscious of the Presence of God, it was my true goal in life. Some months later, in 1985, around February I believe, I went for a consultation with a Clairvoyant for a pain in the neck that was making it increasingly difficult for me to turn my head. I had stopped taking medicine a long time previous because I knew that effects (or illnesses) have a cause and that that cause will pass by means of spiritual uplifting (be it refused or accepted). The benefit of Clairvoyance is that it permits the cause to be understood.

I had already understood so many things about life during those years of searching. But this time, another phase of my progression was going to explode like a nuclear bomb. After the first session, I felt much improved. I did not speak with this woman. She indicated to her Chiropractor colleague the *Chakra* that was not working. He manipulated it very softly and massaged the cervical area. I was very impressed. Then, I returned some weeks later to talk with her. I was already aware of magnetism and manipulation, but I was enraptured by her work and by her presence. I wanted to know more about her. I had felt something as strongly as on the day of my vision. I knew that she was inspired, that she had met God, as I had; she shone with a light like the Angel I had seen.

Without questioning what she told me about my inner life and my present life, I listened as if stunned by truth. She made me live once again what I knew and what I had tried to ignore. Within six months I was transformed, I had given up everything that was unrelated to my quest for a higher self and I followed the advice that she gave. At the beginning of the seventh month, she asked me to prepare to open a healing practice in order to teach Universal Love. I arranged a room to receive the sick and in the months that followed, I renounced everything except the practice of Aikido and of healing. I shut myself off from the outside word and simply read, prayed and meditated.

During this time my friends wondered what was going on. They did not understand the reason for my isolation. God is the essence. We are God's children, to receive a Divine Heritage. They thought I was a fool. Then in May 1987 I left the Ardeche to go to the Pyrennees, to open another practice.

It is now two and a half years since I opened my practice in the town of Mirepoix. During that time I have also been permitted to open a *Dojo* to teach Aikido, to train other

Magnetists, to teach the understanding of the Chakras and of the inner life, and to transform human beings who so wish, into Divine beings. I was drawn to this small town, situated in the centre of a region with a long Spiritual history, through that Clairvoyant who has since become my companion in work and in life. We share our lives and work together for the realisation of others, the realisation of Love on earth.

When first I arrived in this area, I did not know where to start or how I would survive. In one month, I met one person who immediately received the Forces. He spoke to others of what he had seen, and little by little, other people began to come. Then I met a woman who understood my work of laying on hands and the words that I spoke. She lent me her Clinic in the town-centre. The first day I was there, a dog was knocked down by a car. He was in a sorry state and couldn't walk. I took him in my arms and an audience gathered around me. Then I put the dog down and he started to walk again and to bark. I took him up and held him once more, and lo and behold he was healed. I knew then that it would be a good town to work in. Now, under my first-floor apartment, I have a clinic which is open every day to my friends and people from every corner of France, foreigners too.

Opening this clinic was a giant step and I know there are still many more steps for me to take. My Faith in God is reborn each day, my goal is to live here and now in the transparence of the Divine light.

In my work, my main objective is not to treat, or even to heal, illness. My aim is to open the human soul to the direct experience of the Spirit, which is the essence of mankind and is never ill or unhappy. Human beings suffer because of ignorance and a refusal to accept. If we can discover health and trust within ourselves, there is nothing external to fear. There is a Guide, a Master, who directs us; the Father is within each of us. We should therefore understand that each of us has eternal life and that God's Love dwells in each of us. First Commandment: Love God your Father above all else; Second Commandment: Love one another; Third Commandment: Do unto others as thou wouldst be done by.

Spiritual Healing

by Tony Hogan

Tony Hogan *practises Spiritual Healing, Counselling, Absent Healing, Naturopathy, Stress Release, Relaxation therapy, and Hypnotherapy at the Tony Hogan Healing Centre in Kimmage in Dublin.*

The Art of Spiritual Healing has been practised all over the world by different cultures for thousands of years. In every civilisation disease and healing were symbols of profound significance. Illness was seen as the consequences of falling out of Harmony with the Laws of Nature. In order to redress the balance, a reconciliation between man and the forces that govern the pulse of life was necessary, in order to restore him to his full health.

This philosophy is seen in the thinking of all ancient civilisations and is still evident today in those healing traditions that have been handed down through the centuries to the present day. The Greek, Egyptian and Chinese cultures expressed their beliefs in different ways, however they all shared a belief that healing could not be effected purely on a physical level; that it is impossible to separate the spiritual from physical healing, because man exists on a physical, mental and spiritual level. He exists within the universe and the universal energy flows through him, creating his life. It is on this basis that a spiritual healer works, when in some way or another a person is cut off from this free flowing energy which gives life to all aspects of the person's being, and illness is the result.

This same universal energy is known throughout the world as *Ki* to the Japanese, *Prana* to the Hindus, *Chi* to the Chinese, *Mana* to the Polynesians, and *Orenda* to the American Indians. The spiritual healer is a person with a gift which enables him to tap these universal energies and transmit healing to the patient by means of placing his hands on the person, known traditionally as the *laying on of hands*, and in so doing direct a flow of energy to the problem area, thereby increasing the potential for healing to take place.

All healers have different philosophies, beliefs, and use

different approaches with their patients. There are some healers who see themselves as originators of the healing energies, in that they have magnetic personalities and are able to radiate energy and magnetism, these are known as magnetic healers. There are others, namely spiritual healers, who considers themselves as a channel for healing energies which originate from God or Universal Energy and pass through the healer to the patient, affecting him on all levels of his being.

What happens when you go to a Healer?

Normally the healer will sit in front of you, while you tell him/her what the problem is, then he or she will stand either beside you or directly behind you and tune into the source of healing power. Some merely concentrate for a brief moment, others meditate for a while. Then the healer will place his or her hands on the problem area and on the head and transmit healing energy. There are some healers who pass their hands sensitively over the problem area and all over the person keeping their hands a few inches away from the patient's body.

How it feels to have Healing

Each person reacts differently to each healing treatment. Some feel peaceful and warm, some report a relaxed feeling, and a feeling of love. Others experience warmth, still others feel a light tingling sensation like static electricity as the healer's hands pass over the patient's face and head. Others report a feeling of being peaceful and still. However afterwards the patient normally feels calm and relaxed, or energised, for several days.

Recommended Reading
The Power to Heal, by David Harvey (The Aquarian Press).
Healing for You, by Phil Edwards (Thorsons).
The Seven Levels of Healing, by Lila Bek (Rider).
Healing and the Healing Process, by George W. Meek (Quest).
Spiritual and Lay Healing, by Phillippa Pullar (Penguin).

Practitioners

Faith and spirituality play a part in the work of many healers, orthodox and parallel. Those listed below use their hands, or their counsel, in a way that aims to channel healing energies in and to the client. Some spiritual healers have asked not to be listed, preferring people to come to them by other means.

Donegal:
Peter Francis, Meitheal Centre, Inch Fort, Inch Island, Co. Donegal. Tel. 077-60323; Also Rebirthing.

Dublin:
Judith Ashton, 28, Seapoint Ave., Monkstown, Co. Dublin. Tel. 809630. Contact Healing; also, massage, bio-dynamic massage, Reichian bodywork, psychotherapy, counselling, stress-management, Dream Interpretation, energy work; Martin Galvin, 46, Leeson Park, Dublin 6. Tel. 01-604683. Spiritual Healing and Counselling, Psychotherapy and Group Facilitation. Martin works mainly in his clients' homes by appointment; Ida O'Hanlon, Greystones, Co. Wicklow. Tel. 01-875397. Healing, in particular the areas of Kinesiology, Reflexology and the Metamorphic Technique. Her main orientation is now to energy healing.

Centres

The Healing House, 24, O'Connell Ave., off Berkeley Rd., Dublin 7. Tel. 306413. Joseph Hoey: Laying on of hands. Also Hypnotherapy and Nutritional Counselling; John Kenny: Spiritual Psychotherapeutics.

Tony Hogan Healing Centre, 11, Sundrive Road, Kimmage, Dublin 12. Tel. 01-906504. Also Counselling, Absent Healing, Naturopathy, Stress release and relaxation therapy, Hypnotherapy, Self Healing.

Bio-Healing

Bio-healing became widely known in Ireland in early 1990 when two practitioners appeared on RTE's *Late Late Show*. Bio-healing combines a scientific approach with work on the energy field around the body. It is a new and exciting development and is undergoing further research in this country and elsewhere. For further information and appointments tel. 094-81402.

Courses

Courses in Spiritual Psychotherapy are run from time to time by Peter and Elizabeth Gill of The Way Mark Centre, The Old

Rectory, Dunganstown, Wicklow, Co. Wicklow. Tel. 0404-7220 between 10am and 6pm for further information.

IAHM Healing Therapists (trained by Tony Quinn) See p. 217.

Cork:
Imelda Farrell RGN RM MYogaTher, Tony Quinn Healing Therapy, 20 Academy St., Cork; Peadar Cox DHN, Tony Quinn Centre, 20 Academy St., Cork. Tel. 021-276364; Jenny Dolan BSc DHPM DHN, Beausite, Rushbrooke, Cobh, Co. Cork. Tel. 021-812218; Liam Woods DHPM, 9 Trabeg Ave., Douglas. Tel. 021-276364.

Louth:
Thomas Dolan DHPM MIAHM, Tony Quinn Centre, 18 Jocelyn St., Dundalk, Co. Louth.

Wicklow:
Tom McKenna DHN MIAHM, Tony Quinn Healing Therapy, Bray; Brendan Clifford DHN MIAHM, Tony Quinn Centre, Bray.

Dublin County — South:
Paul Doyle DHPM DHN MIAHM, 3 Avondale Lawn Est., Blackrock, Co. Dublin. Tel. 887432; Bernard Kelly DHPM MIAHM, 5 Mather Road Sth., Mount Merrion, Co. Dublin. Tel. 886905; John Brerton DHPM MIAHM, 8 Mountdown Park, Dun Loaghaire, Co. Dublin. Tel. 800512.

Dublin 6:
Martin O'Neill DHPM MIAHM, Tony Quinn Centre, 2 Wynnfield Rd., Rathmines, Dublin 6; Patricia McNally BComm MYogaTher MIAHM, Tony Quinn Healing Therapy, 2 Wynnfield Rd., Rathmines; Also at: Tony Quinn Healing Therapy, Dun Laoghaire; Mary Howick DHPM MIAHM, 54 Lr. Beechwood Ave., Ranelagh, Dublin 6. Tel. 688355w, 962371h.

Dublin 16:
Anne Kelleher BA DHPM MIAHM, 27, Glenvara Park, Ballycullen Road, Templeogue, Dublin 16. Tel. 942178.

Dublin 18:
Margaret Crehan DHPM MIAHM, 1 Hainault Lawn, Foxrock, Dublin 18. Tel. 894779.

Dublin 20:
Margaret Glover DHPM MIAHM, 65 Kennelsfort Rd., Palmerstown, Dublin 20. Tel. 269142.

North Dublin — Dublin 3:
Margaret Forde BH HDipEd DipApPsych MIAHM, Tony Quinn Healing Therapy, 316 Howth Rd., Dublin 3; Joan Gleeson BH DHPM MIAHM, 61 Seapark Drive, Clontarf, Dublin 3. Tel. 331917; Catherine Gleeson BA DHPM MIAHM, 50 Seapark, Mt. Prospect Ave., Clontarf, Dublin 3. Tel. 334025.

Dublin 7:
Tony Quinn DHM MIAHM, c/o 66 Eccles St. (Residential seminars only); Aideen Cowman, MYogaTher MIAHM, Tony Quinn Healing Therapy, 66 Eccles St., Dublin 7. Tel. 304078; Patricia McNally BComm MYogaTher MIAHM, Tony Quinn Healing Therapy, 66 Eccles St., Dublin 7; Tom McKenna DHN MIAHM, Tony Quinn Healing Therapy, 66 Eccles St., Dublin 7; Martin Forde BA ND MRN DO MRO MIAHM, Tony Quinn Centre, 66 Eccles St., Dublin 7; Tom Carter DHPM MIAHM, Tony Quinn Centre, 66 Eccles St., Dublin 7. Tel. 304078; Hugh Chambers DHN MIAHM, Tony Quinn

Centre, 66 Eccles St., Dublin 7; Dympna Lynch DHPM MIAHM, 22 Shandon Road, Phisboro, Dublin 7. Tel. 303715; Enda McDonnell BEng DHPM MIAHM, 3 Nelson St., Dublin 7. Tel. 308658.

Dublin 9:
Bernie Brannick DHPM MIAHM, 151 Celtic Park Ave., Whitehall, Dublin 9. Tel. 314967.

Dublin 15:
Tom McKenna DHN MIAHM, Tony Quinn Healing Therapy, 10 Park Drive Grove, Castleknock.

Chapter Thirteen

Information on AIDS and HIV Positive

Human Immunodeficiency Virus (HIV) is a virus that attacks the human immune system, making it difficult for the body to fight off infections. There are four ways that the virus can be transmitted from one person to another:
— through the exchange of bodily fluids (semen or vaginal fluids) during sexual intercourse;
— through the sharing of used needles and syringes among intravenous drug users;
— through the transfusion of blood and blood products (in this country all blood is screened for HIV);
— from a woman who is HIV positive to her child before or during birth or possibly through breastfeeding.

HIV **cannot** be spread through everyday contact with someone who is HIV positive or has AIDS, or through kissing, hugging, sharing crockery or cutlery, or through living with someone who has AIDS. Although many people are fearful that they may catch the virus from a person who is infected, many of our fears are based on misinformation received through the media.

In Ireland, there are 969 people known to be infected with the HIV virus (August 1990). These people have all had a special blood test which searches for the antibodies that have been created in the blood system to the HIV. These people have all had positive test results and now know that they have been in contact with the virus. It is essential that anyone considering taking this test discusses their decision with a counsellor before doing so. There are many reasons for this:
— people may have been misinformed about modes of transmission and may need to reconsider whether or not their behaviour has put them at risk of coming in contact with the virus;

— the person taking the test needs to carefully consider how they might react to either a positive or negative result. A positive result will obviously be difficult. Many may still have questions or need extra information about protecting themselves from possible exposure to the virus even if they get a negative result;

— simply taking the test (regardless of the result) may have long-term implications for individuals who are seeking life assurance or mortgages.

Test results should be given in person rather than over the phone in order to give the individual the opportunity to discuss any queries they may have.

Of the 969 individuals diagnosed with HIV, 157 have gone on to develop AIDS and 68 have died. *Acquired Immune Deficiency Syndrome* ('AIDS') is diagnosed in people who are HIV positive only after they have been ill with an opportunistic infection, an infection that would only occur because the person's immune system has been suppressed by the HIV. Some of these infections include *PCP* (a type of pneumonia), *KS* (a type of cancer), cytomeglovirus etc. Many of these illnesses are, of themselves, treatable and many people with AIDS can return to an acceptable level of health. While people with AIDS may not feel 100% healthy all the time, many continue to work and get on with their lives generally. It is only at the terminal stages of their illness, when the body has lost most of its ability to fight off infections that the person may need long bouts of time in a hospital bed or being cared for at home. The length of time that each individual lives with AIDS differs and with new drugs being developed, this length of time is being constantly extended.

With a current rate of increase that is the highest in Europe with the number of AIDS cases doubling every 10 months, we cannot remain removed from this problem in this country. While we would hope never to reach the numbers predicted by the Minister for Health in May 1989 of 12,000 cases of AIDS by 1995, this virus will both infect and affect many more people in the years to come. Prevention is obviously better than a cure and it is not just those who are HIV positive who should consider changing behaviour that puts them at risk of being

HIV positive. For those who are already infected, access to a good quality, and an understanding, health service is essential while more understanding from the community at large could eliminate some of the isolation experienced by those who are HIV positive or have AIDS.

Centres
Dublin:
AIDS Action Alliance
Cairde; Body Positive; Practical Aid; Frontliners Ireland; Gay Health Action; Women and AIDS: all at Avoca House, Parnell Street, Dublin 1. Tel. 733799.
AIDS Fund
13 Upper Ormond Quay, Dublin 7.

Cork:
Cork AIDS Alliance, 16 Peters Street, Cork. Tel. 021-275837.

Galway:
Western AIDS Alliance, Uzanam House, St. Augustine Street, Galway. Tel. 091-66266.

Support Services for HIV Drug Users
Dublin:
Anna Liffey Project, 13 Lr. Abbey Street, Dublin 1. Tel. 786899/786828; Youth Action Project Ballymun, 4 Balcurris Road, Ballymun, Dublin 11. Tel. 428071; Drug Treatment Centre Board, Trinity Court, Pearse Street, Dublin 2. Tel. 771122; AIDS Resource Centre, 19 Haddington Road, Dublin 4. Tel. 602149; Coolmine House, 19 Lord Edward Street, Dublin 2. Tel. 782300.

AIDS Helplines
Dublin:
AIDS Helpline Dublin, P.O. Box 1884, Dublin 1. Tel. 724277; Mon. - Fri. 7 - 9 p.m./Sat. 3 - 6 p.m.; AIDS Phone-in Service, tel. 838677; Tues. 2 - 5 p.m./Thurs. 7 - 9 p.m.

Cork:
AIDS Helpline Cork, tel. 021-276676; Mon. and Thurs. 7 - 9 p.m./Sat. 2 - 6 p.m.

Galway:
AIDS Helpline Galway, tel. 091-64000; Tues. 10 a.m. - 1 p.m., 2 - 4 p.m./Wed. 10 a.m. - 1 p.m.; Western AIDS Alliance Helpline, tel. 091-66266; Thurs. 8 - 10 p.m.

Northern Ireland:
AIDS Helpline Belfast, P.O. Box 206, Belfast BT1 1SJ. Tel. 084-326117; Mon., Wed., Fri. 7.30 - 10 p.m./Sat. 2 - 5 p.m.

STD Clinics
Dublin:
St. James' Hospital G U Clinic, Hospital 5, Dublin 8. Tel. 535245 (by appointment only); Mater Hospital STD Clinic, Out Patients Department, North Circular Road, Dublin 7. Tel. 01-304488 during clinic times, 01-301995 (main hospital); Male: Wed. and Thurs. 4 - 7 p.m., Female: Tues. 4 - 7 p.m./Thur. 3 - 4 p.m.; Victoria Hospital Cork, Infirmary Road, Cork. Tel. 021-966844; Mon. 5.30 - 7 p.m./Wed. 10 a.m. - 12 noon; Western Health Board, tel. 091-64000 (by appointment); Limerick Regional Hospital, Dooradoyle. Tel. 061-28111; Fri. 2.30 - 4.30 p.m. only; Royal Victoria Hospital, Falls Road, Belfast. Tel. 084-320159 during clinic hours; Mon. - Fri. 9 - 11 a.m.; Mon., Wed., Fri. 2 - 3 p.m.; Altnagelvin Hospital, Derry. Tel. 080504-47257; Mon., Tues., Wed., Fri. 9.30 - 10.30 p.m.

Sexuality Switchboards
Dublin:
Gay Switchboard Dublin, 13 Christchurch Place, Dublin 8. Tel. 01-721055; Mon. - Fri. 8 - 10 p.m., Sat. 3.30 - 6 p.m., Sun. 7 - 9 p.m.; Lesbian Line. Tel. 01-613777; Thurs. 7 - 9 p.m.; Act, Adolescent Confidential Telephone, Service for young people. Tel. 01-740723/744133; Sat. 1 - 5 p.m.

Cork:
Gay Information Cork, tel. 021-317026; Wed. 7 - 9 p.m.; Lesbian Line Cork, tel. 021-317023; Thur. 8 - 10 p.m.;

Gay/Lesbian Line Galway, tel. 091-24810; Wed. 8 - 10 p.m.;
Gay/Lesbian Line Limerick, tel. 061-310101; Mon. 7 - 8.30
p.m. (Men); Thur. 7 - 8.30 p.m. (Women); Cara-Friend Belfast,
tel. 084-322023; Mon., Tue., Wed. 7.30 - 10 p.m.; Lesbian Line
Belfast, tel. 084-238668; Thur. 8 - 10 p.m.; Belfast Gay/Lesbian
Drop-in Centre, Cathedral Buildings, Lower Donegal Street,
Belfast. Sat. 1.30 - 5 p.m.; Cara-Friend Derry, tel. 080504-
263120; Thurs. 7.30 - 10 p.m. Lesbians 1st and 3rd Thurs.

DIRECTORY

Alternative Healing Centres, Organisations, Publications, Suppliers of Natural Medicines

Centres

Antrim:

Lifespring, 111, Cliftonville Rd., Belfast BT14. Tel. 0232-753658. Lifespring is established without distinction of sex, race, political or religious opinions. It offers individual counselling sessions; individual Aromatherapy consultations with nutritional guidance and relaxation exercises.

Workshops and courses on offer include: Art for All; Creative Writing; Personal Growth through journalling; Relationships — the Family of Origin approach to gaining selfhood; Aromatherapy for partners and friends; Aromatherapy workshops for handicapped children and their carers; Personal Effectiveness Courses; Developmental Psychology; Weekly Meditation groups; Lifespring Retreats; 'Time for Me' for women in conjunction with University of Ulster.

Mary Grant, the Co-ordinator of Lifespring has worked in a voluntary professional capacity in West Belfast since 1972. She initiated and guided the establishment of the Ardoyne Family Centre and the Christian Life Communities; and in 1981, the Cornerstone Community, in 1987, Lifespring. She also runs an Aromatherapy training centre and practise.

Some of the people who regularly offer services at

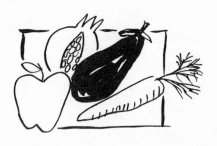

Lifespring include: Kate McVeigh — Aromatherapy; Margaret McMackin — Counselling; Deirdre Kennedy — Counselling and courses including co-counselling; Brendan Kennedy — Counselling and Developmental Psychology; Martin Donnelly — Counselling: Transpersonal Perspective; Mary Moran — Management, Personal Effectiveness; Patricia Gore — Art for All — Adults and children and Creative Writing; Lily Williams — Encourages new writers; Facilitators who visit regularly include: Mike Cowan — From the US on Selfhood, Mutuality, and Family-of-Origin themes; Ian Gordon Brown and others on Transpersonal Psychology; Institute of Marriage and Family Therapy — Systems approach to Family Therapy; Angela Walsh — Family Reconstruction; Helen Johnson and Paul Nemeer — Voice Development and many other creative possibilities; Liz Comerton — Yoga and her 'Look Good, Feel Good' programme; Joe Boyle — Results Workshop; Corporate Financial Services on Money Management.

Clare:

Cooleenbridge Community Co-operative Society Limited, Main Street, Scariff, Co. Clare. Tel. 0619-21265.

The Co-op is a development agency in rural East Clare providing support to its members and their enterprises. These enterprises which are separated legally and financially from the Co-op, include a wholefood shop, puppet theatre group and organic paint suppliers. The Co-op intends to research and support the establishment of further commercial enterprises providing long term employment for its members. These enterprises will be based on the need to develop socially useful goods and services which are ecologically sustainable.

Cork:

Rainbow Health Centre, Rainbow House, Derrycreha, Glengarriff, Co. Cork. Tel. 027-63019.

At the Rainbow Health Centre, Francis Quinton offers the following range of therapies: Chiropractic, Medical Massage, Rolfing, Homoeopathy, Counselling and Psychotherapy. Francis Quinton holds West German State Degrees and Diplomas in these therapies.

Tony Quinn Centre, 20 Academy St., Cork. Tel. 021-276364.

Health Store; Healing Therapy; Ki Masage; Holistic Nutrition; Diploma courses in Holistic Medicine. See p. 212.

Donegal:

Meitheal Centre, Inch Island, Co. Donegal. Tel. Buncrana 077-60323.

Meitheal (Irish for co-operative working group) is a spiritual community and holistic education centre on the shores of Lough Swilly, about 10 miles west of Derry. The community was founded in 1986 and the Meitheal Trust owns a five acre property which includes three houses, a meditation sanctuary, organic gardens, a pier and an old British navy fort. Members are self-supporting and practice a variety of healing therapies and crafts. Their activities are based on personal and group meditation, regular sharings and concensus decision making. They run guest programmes, workshops, gatherings and family summer camps, produce a bi-annual newsletter (at Easter and Christmas), and grow organic fruit and vegetables. To receive their newsletter or other information write to the address above.

Dublin:

Amethyst Resources for Human Development. Tel. 01-862428.

Amethyst is a resource for human development with a body-mind-spirit approach to health and healing, and a belief that society and the planet can be healed if we start with ourselves. Amethyst offers individual assessments, healing and therapy sessions; workshops and training programmes for those interested in learning practical healing techniques for themselves and others; intensive primal integration and regression therapy; meditation and visualisation for healing and personal growth. From time to time visiting experts from elsewhere teach at Amethyst. A feature of the annual programme is the experiential summer school which will be held in Ireland and in England in 1990. A healing clinic which anyone may attend is held weekly (apart from Bank Holiday weekends) on a Friday night at Dunstaffnage, St. Brigid's Church Rd., Stillorgan, Co. Dublin between 7 and 9 pm. This is staffed by advanced trainees in the healing programme.

Further information may be obtained from: Alison Hunter, Curtlestown, Enniskerry, Co. Wicklow. Tel. 01-862428. She founded Amethyst in 1981 and is a skilled and experienced group leader and regression therapist.

Her co-partner, Shirley Ward MEd DipED MFPhys is a member of the AHP Practitioners, has a Master's degree in Education and an international qualification in massage. She is now a director of Amethyst, counselling and healing people with stress related illnesses.

Dublin Food Co-op, Carmichael House, Brunswick St., Dublin 1. Tel. 01-721191.

Dublin Food Co-op is a consumer's wholefood co-op. Its consumer members wholly co-own, control, operate and consume the goods and services provided by their joint efforts. The Co-op was established in January 1983 with the aim of making shopping an amiable, communal experience and to make available to its members, organically grown and natural wholefoods at wholesale prices. The Co-op is open fortnightly on Saturdays at St. Andrew's Community Centre, Pearse St., Dublin 2. Further information is available from the above address.

John Rogers Natural Health Training Centre, 1, Park Lane East (Rear 206, Pearse St.), Dublin 2. Tel. 01-718545.

Classes in Aikido, Yoga, Makko Ho, Shi and Stretch. Van Key Vacuum Cupping treatment, a method for improving and restoring health by enhancing blood quality and circulation. Particularly effective in the treatment of Fibrisitis, Rheumatism, Sports Injuries, persistent coughs. John Rogers also gives dietary advice in conjunction with massage.

Kiltalown House, Jobstown, Tallaght, Dublin 24. Tel. 01-522466.

Kiltalown House is an 18th century house in Jobstown, Tallaght, where a centre was established in 1987 by a group of local people. The main aim of the Centre is to provide the opportunity to empower the whole person through developing their creativity.

Activities: Youth Club; Aromatherapy, Yoga and Coun-selling with Imelda Doyle; Osteopathy with Chris Campbell;

Wholefood Cooking with Veronica Crombie; Creating and Reflecting with Jo O'Connell, 2nd Sunday of every month; Circle Dancing Creativity, Creation Centred Spirituality, Circle Dancing with Imelda Smyth; Relaxation/Meditation, Communication Skills and Yoga with Jane Duncan; Co-Counselling and Personal Development with Maeve Dunne; Reflexology with Patricia Swann; Shiatsu; Voice/Clowning; I Can't Draw; Enneagram. Please ring to make an appointment.

The Natural Living Centre, 5, St. James' Terrace, Malahide, Co. Dublin. Tel. 01-452050.

The Natural Living Centre opened in April '89 to promote the growth of Complementary Therapies and Natural Healing. Courses and classes: workshops, weekends and daily treatments are provided.

Courses and Classes: Yoga with Phil Brady; Tai Chi Chuan with Joe Hoey; Shiatsu with Joe Maguire; Natural Healing — Self Healing with Joe Hoey; Astrology with Terri Blanche; Diploma Courses in Holistic Massage, Aromatherapy and Reflexology with Roisin Hilliard and Phil Brady.

Workshops: Workshops conducted by visiting authorities include drawing for inner development; Crystal Therapy; Body Harmony; Aromatherapy; Shiatsu; Astrology.

Daily Treatments: Holistic Massage with Roisin Hilliard, Phil Brady and Joe Hoey; Aromatherapy with Roisin Hilliard and Phil Brady; Reflexology with Mary Lyons; Astrology with Terri Blanche; Natural Healing with Joe Hoey.

The Source, 11 East Essex St., Dublin 2.

The Source is a centre which sells essential tools for self development and offers a facility for meditation and healing sessions. Masta, Rohit and Jaya lead meditations, run workshops on intuition and art, and use crystals in healing work. Introductory workshops on many of the healing arts will take place here. A programme of meditations and workshops is available.

Teach Bán, 6, Parnell Road, Harolds Cross, Dublin 6. Tel. 01-543943.

Ann Currie and Patrick Duggan teach and practise alternative medicine basing their work on the principles and practise of Shiatsu and Macrobiotics. Classes are offered in Shiatsu, Wholefood Cookery, Alternative/Oriental Medicine. Beginners and more advanced classes are provided.

Tony Quinn Centre, 66 Eccles St., Dublin 7. Tel. 303717/301154; 2 Winnefield Rd., Rathmines, Dublin 6. Tel. 01-974234; 96 Lr. George's St., Dun Laoghaire, Dublin. Tel. 01-809891.

Health Store; Healing Therapy; Ki Massage; Holistic Nutrition. Diploma courses in Holistic Medicine. See also p. 217.

Turning Point, 2, Lansdowne Gardens, Shelbourne Rd., Dublin 4. Tel. 01-602600/680568.

Turning Point is a holistic health centre offering support, through a range of services, to those facing crises and life-threatening illnesses such as cancer, AIDS and bereavement. The holistic programme of healing offered by Turning Point includes counselling/psychotherapy, autogenic training, dietary advice, homoeopathic medicine, acupuncture, visualisation and assertiveness training. It is designed to help people in overcoming stress, coping with crises and strengthening the immune system to combat physical disease. Turning Point also offers an annual programme of workshops, copies of which are available on request. Highlight of the year is the 'Life, Death and Transition' workshop organised by Turning Point for the Elizabeth Kubler-Ross Centre in the US.

The Turning Point team consists of: Kay Conroy, Autogenic trainer, founder-director, administrator and therapist at Turning Point. Clare Counihan, peer counsellor, Family Therapist and Gestalt Therapist; Kathleen Dillon, who worked as a Cancer Research Chemist in Brandels University, Boston, and has training in Marriage Counselling and Gestalt Therapy; Kay Ferriter, who has a special interest in the issues affecting people who have grown up in addicted families; Celine Leonard, a Counsellor and practitioner of Five Element Acupuncture; Dr. Elizabeth Ogden, a practitioner of alternative and complementary disciplines focusing mainly on homoeopathy, diet and acupuncture; Catherine O'Dea, who is a social worker and has worked with women individually and in groups; Delma O'Regan worked as a medical social worker for 10 years with those going through the crisis of surgery, chronic illness, terminal illness, bereavement and birth of a handicapped child; Mary Paula Walsh, a founder-director, co-ordinator and senior therapist at Turning Point.

Galway:
Slanu, Galway Cancer Help Centre. Tel. 091-55023.

Slanu means being saved, redeemed, made whole; being led out of bondage and oppression into freedom and fullness of life. Slanu offers a programme of supportive therapies for people with a cancer diagnosis, and preventative programmes which are open to all. Slanu's philosophy is holistic — that there needs to be harmony between body, mind and spirit if we are to grow towards wholeness and to live fully. The programmes include individual counselling, journalling, art therapy, autogenics/relaxation/visualisation, nutritional and medical consultation, guidelines for healthy eating, healing prayer, meditation. The programme addresses the needs of the whole person in an atmosphere of care and concern. It is intended as a complement to orthodox methods of surgery, radio/chemotherapy and on-going medical care. The programme is staffed by qualified personnel including counsellors, psychologist, doctor, dietitian, spiritual helper. The programme is residential and is held on the first and third weeks of every month. The meals served are Vegan, i.e. no dairy produce, meat, fish, poultry, tea or coffee. Clients are asked to contribute according to their ability to pay and Slanu is primarily dependent on sponsorship, donations and fundraising.

Kerry:
Lios Dana, Natural Living Centre, Inch, Co. Kerry. Tel. Ann Hyland, Michael Travers, 066-58189.

Lios Dana is a residential holistic retreat providing a wide range of facilities, activities and courses. Facilities include weekend or weekly accommodation, Vegetarian, Macrobiotic and Seafood meals, visits to archaeological sites and ancient stone monuments, contact with local arts and crafts. Activities include Yoga, meditation, cooking, outdoor activities. Classes are held either as evening classes or as part of a course in art, Aikido, Shiatsu-Acupressure. Discussion of diet, nutrition and natural health care may be included in weekend programmes for those who request it. Copies of the 1990 programme and prices are available on request. The facilities of the centre are also available for hire by groups and organisations who wish to hold seminars and workshops.

The Signal Box Health Farm Glenbeigh, Co. Kerry. Tel. 066-68240.

The Signal Box offers Health Diets; Health Care; Gymnastics; Yoga; Chiropody; Sauna; Solarium; Workout-Room and specialises in the Schroth (Dry-Diet) Treatment. The treatment normally runs for three weeks and can be modified to cater for individual needs.

Louth:
Iomlanu Centre for Healing and Creative Living, 36, Castle Road, Dundalk. Tel. 042-32804.

Iomlanu is the Irish word for wholeness and fulfillment. The aim of the Centre is to provide people with a place and opportunity to tap into their inner resources and wisdom, heal the hurts and wounds within themselves, learn ways of reducing stress in daily life, explore ways of living with greater awareness and responsibility and happiness and in harmony with self, nature and God. Workshops and seminars are held regularly and a programme is available from the Centre. Creation Centred Spirituality gatherings are held monthly. The following services are also available at Iomlanu: Reflexology with Roisin Carroll; Stress Management and Nutritional Advice with Ann Marie McGlinchey; Massage and Healing with Dolores Whelan; Shiatsu with Anne Finn; Homoeopathy with Olli Kelly; Psychotherapy and Stress Counselling with Brian McNamee; Massage with Kristan O'Donovan.

Tony Quinn Centre, 18 Jocelyn St., Dundalk. Tel. 042-38097.

Health Store; Healing Therapy; Ki Massage; Holistic

Nutrition. Diploma courses in Holistic Medicine. See also p. 217.

Mayo:
Cloona Health Centre, Westport, Co. Mayo. Tel. 098-25251.

Cloona Health Centre offers week-long residential courses from March to October. The programme is primarily a cleansing course, with a strong emphasis on relaxation and exercise. There is no smoking in Cloona, and no tea or coffee, but a wide selection of herb teas. Breakfast, Lunch and Supper are served daily and a Sauna and massage are available in the evening. Contact : Emer Gaffney for details.

Monaghan:
Tony Quinn Centre, 22 O'Neill St., Carrickmacross, Co. Monaghan. Tel. 042-61680.

Health Store; Healing Therapy; Ki Massage; Holistic Nutrition. Diploma courses in Holistic Medicine. See also p. 212.

Wicklow:
The Hermitage Centre for the Healing Arts, Newtownmountkennedy, Co. Wicklow. Tel. Judith Crowe or David Marshall 01-819515.

The Hermitage is developing as a centre for the healing arts. The seminar room accommodates up to 25 people and is available for workshops and groups. Self-catering facilities are provided, or vegetarian home-cooked food can be provided. Weekend workshops on personal development, rebirthing, Yoga and related interests are offered.

Tony Quinn Centre, 1 Mill Lane, Bray, Co. Wicklow. Tel. 01-869311.

Health Store; Healing Therapy; Ki Massage; Holistic Nutrition. Diploma courses in Holistic Medicine.

Organisations

The Irish Holistic Health Association (IHHA)

The IHHA was founded in 1982. It promotes changes in lifestyle through various disciplines such as Shiatsu, Aikido, wholefood cooking, Yoga, meditation and other holistic ways of living. The holistic approach to health sees the inter-relationship between body, mind and spirit and emphasises the need to live in harmony with the environment. Seminars and workshops are regularly organised with both visiting teachers and members of the Association. Membership is open and an annual general meeting is held each December.

The IHHA has a general membership throughout the 32 counties, and members who practice a range of therapies including Aikido; Aromatherapy; Shiatsu; Osteopathy; Reflexology; and T'ai Chi Ch'uan. Workshops in all of the major centres are planned during the coming months, enquiries are welcome. A list of IHHA practitioners and membership application forms are available from The Secretary, the IHHA, 23, Viking Road, Arbour Hill, Dublin 7. Tel. 01-772058. Individual membership costs £12 per annum, the household/group fee is £18 per annum.

Tony Quinn Centres

Tony Quinn began to teach Yoga in Ireland in 1971. He had researched health, healing, self and life improvements, physical culture and philosophy and went on to found centres where his philosophy of Holistic Medicine is applied. The basic principle of the Tony Quinn philosophy is that 'there is an underlying life force or energy which is available to each person. The purpose of Holistic Medicine is to unite the person with their inner source of this life-force or energy'.

Therapies available are Healing Therapy, Ki Massage Therapy and Holistic Nutrition. Postal Requests; Healing Therapy can be carried out by writing or calling to The President, IHAC, 66 Eccles St., Dublin 7.

The Irish Association of Holistic Medicine (IAHM) was founded in 1986 by a group of Holistic practitioners from the Tony Quinn Centres. The IAHM offers qualifications as follows. All qualifications require a minimum of three years' training including in all cases Philosophy, Psychotherapy and Dietetics:

DHPM: (Diploma in Holistic Preventive Medicine). These members may specialise in Ki Massage, Yoga, Ki Exercises, in Psychotherapy of Healing therapy.

DHD: (Diploma in Holistic Dietetics). All holders are qualified in Clinical Nutrition.

M. Yoga Ther.: (A Master diploma in Yoga Therapy). Awarded on the basis of proven ability rather than examination results alone.

DHM: (Diploma in Holistic Medicine). Only those who fulfil the requirements for the DHPM and the DHN are eligible.

The Irish Health Culture Association

Founded in 1968 by Tony Quinn as the Irish Physical Culture Association, later expanded into the much broader field of Health Culture, which is essentially a form of preventative medicine. The minimum requirement for membership is a diploma from a one-year part-time course. The IHCA courses are Ki Massage, Holistic Dietetics, and Yoga, and all are based on the Holistic Principle. Membership is renewed yearly by subscription. Members are bound by a code of ethics and undergo practice inspection. Continuing education is obligatory. Members may take out Professional Indemnity Insurance via the Association group scheme. The prospectus of the IHCA and IAHM is available by writing or calling to The President, IHCA, 66, Eccles St., Dublin 7.

The Metamorphic Association

The Metamorphic Technique is a method of self-healing and creative growth. It does not involve a treatment of particular symptoms, but brings about movement of old patterns of illness, both physical and psychological, and helps the individual to evolve. Monthly meetings are held in Fermoy, Dundalk, Dublin and Cork. The Metamorphic Association produces a membership list of those qualified to teach and apply the technique to others.

Books and tapes are also available from the Association at either of the following addresses: 27, Meadow Grove, Blackrock, Cork. Tel. 021-357566; 12, Glandore Park, Monkstown, Co. Dublin. Tel. 01-806104.

The Kinesiology Institute

Kinesiology is a science of muscle-testing, discovered and researched by Dr. George Goodheart DC in America in the 1960s. In Kinesiology, muscles are tested in a gentle way and if they are found to be weak, then special reflex points on the body are stimulated in order to restore normal lymph, blood or nerve circulation or flow of Chi. Introductory courses in Kinesiology are provided by the Kinesiology Institute. The courses are known as Touch For Health. The introductory course is of 3 weekends, duration, and is suitable for professionals and lay people who wish to use Kinesiology among friends and family. Further information about courses and practitioners is available from : Risteard de Barra, Secretary, The Kinesiology Institute, 84, Cappaghmore, Clondalkin, Dublin 22. Tel. 01-571183.

Retail outlets stocking natural medicines

Dublin:
Ballinteer Pharmacy, Dublin. Burkes Pharmacy, Glasthule Rd., Dun Laoghaire. Ceres, Powerscourt Townhouse. Cleary's, O'Connell St., Dublin. Cornucopia, Wicklow St., Dublin. Crowley Pharmacy, Superquinn Centre, Blackrock. Crowley Pharmacy, 6, Lower Baggot St., Dublin. Crowley Homoeopathic Pharmacy, Nassau St., Dublin 2. The Country Cellar, Patrick St., Dun Laoghaire. Doran Pharmacy, Crazy Prices Centre, Ballybrack. Down to Earth, Georges St., Dublin. Eason's O'Connell St., Dublin. Farmers Pharmacy, Dundrum Shopping Centre. Foley, M.P.S.I., Parnell St., Dublin. General Health Food Store, Marlborough St., Dublin. The Grape'n'Grain, The Triangle, Ranelagh. Granny's Kitchen, The Arcade, Main St., Dundrum. Hayes, Coyningham Robinson, Grafton St. Hayes, Coyningham, Nutgrove Centre, Rathfarnham. The Hopsack, The Swan Centre, Rathmines. Kenn's Chemist, Dalkey. Lallo M.P.S.I., Phibsboro. Leonards' Corner Pharmacy, South Circular Road. Lynham Pharmacy, Knocklyon Shopping Centre. Morehampton Pharmacy, Morehampton Rd. Murphy Pharmacy, Talbot St. Murray's Chemist, Killiney. Murray's Chemist, Stillorgan Shopping Centre. Murray's Pharmacy, Roches Stores Centre Blackrock. Nature's Way, Superquinn Centre, Blackrock. Nature's Way, Ilac Centre. Nature's Way, Stephen's Green Centre. Nolan's Pharmacy, Glenageary, Co. Dublin. Nunane Pharmacy, Bellvue Ace., Glenageary. The Nutkeg, Castle Centre, Swords. O'Connell's Pharmacy, O'Connell Street. O'Connells Pharmacy, 310 Harold's Cross Rd. O'Farrell's Pharmacy, Artane Shopping Centre. Rafferty Pharmacy, Stillorgan Shopping Centre. Rafferty Pharmacy, Dunnes Stores, Cornelscourt. R.N.J. Pharmacy, Donaghmede. Travers Pharmacy, 8, The Mall, Donnybrook. Walsh's Pharmacy, Rathfarnham Shopping Centre.

Connaught/Ulster:
W.S.Black, Mill St., Monaghan. C.J. Farren, Main St., Buncrana, Co. Donegal. Feely M.P.S.I., Tuam, Co. Galway. Golden M.P.S.I., Westport, Co. Mayo. Hayes and Hayes Pharmacy, Portumna. Albert Hanberry, Ennis Co. Clare. Nature's Work, Market Square, Monaghan. Heneghan M.P.S.I.,,, Castlebar, Co. Mayo. Healthwise, Lr. Abbeygate St., Galway. The Honey Pot, Irishtown, Athlone. Honeycomb, Upr. Abbeygate St., Galway. McHadden M.P.S.I., Letterkenny. Mulreaney M.P.S.I., Sligo. Natural Way, 47a, Lower Main St., Letterkenny. O'Sullivan, Newcastlewest. Simple Simon, Main St., Donegal.

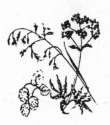

North Leinster:

Brownes Pharmacy, Coothill, Co. Cavan. Clones Pharmacy, Clones, Co. Monaghan. Corcoran's Chemist, Main Street, Longford. Peter Kavanagh, Dunshaughlin, Co. Meath. Mathews Pharmacy, Boyne Centre, Drogheda. Mathews Pharmacy, Ardee. Next to Nature, Brewer's Hill, Navan, Co. Meath. Nuts'n'Grains, Mullingar, Co. Westmeath. Town Centre Pharmacy, Drogheda.

South Leinster:

Beatha Health Foods, Liberty Sq., Thurles. Butlers Medical Hall, Main St., Wicklow. Connolly's Chemists, 59, Main St., Dungarvan, Co. Waterford. The Dargle Pharmacy, Dargle Shopping Centre, Bray. Declan Dowling, Waterford. Sandra Duffy, Arklow, Co. Wicklow. Fruit and Nut Place, Portlaoise. Full of Beans, Georges Court, Waterford. Fogarty, Kilmallock. Friary Pharmacy, Thurles, Co. Tipperary. Good Inside, 12, Charles St., New Ross. Good Earth, Kieran St., Kilkenny. The Honey Pot, Tullow House, Carlow. A Humble Natural Food Shop, Rowe Street, Wexford. Kinsella M.P.S.I., Edenderry Co. Offaly. Madden Pharmacy, Athy. McCauley M.P.S.I., Gorey, Co. Wexford. Mc Cauley M.P.S.I., Enniscorthy, Co. Wexford. Nature's Remedies, Michael St., Waterford. Nature's Gold, 1, Killincarrig Rd., Greystones. The Nutkeg, Quinsborough Centre, Bray. Michael O'Connell Pharmacy, High St. Kilkenny. Only Natural, Lower Main St., Wexford. Young M.P.S.I., Newbridge, Co. Kildare. Walsh M.P.S.I., Celbridge, Co. Kildare.

Munster:

Bandon Medical Hall, Bridge St., Bandon, Cork. Cassidy's Pharmacy, William St., Limerick. Cassidy's Pharmacy, Crescent Centre, Limerick. Coen, Bantry. Crowley's Pharmacy, Market Square, Dunmanway. Sean Collins Pharmacy, Killaloe, Co. Clare. Finbar Dalton, Ballincollig, Cork. Duffy M.P.S.I., Cork. Eats of Eden, Lower Cecil St., Limerick. Falvey Pharmacy, 33, Douglas Shopping Centre, Cork. Dermot Foley, Limerick. French, New Ross, Co. Wexford. The Grove, Upr. Cecil St., Limerick. Hayes Coyningham Robinson, Wilton Centre, Cork. The Honey Pot, Michael St., Clonmel. McCann's, Tralee, Co. Kerry. McGuire's, Listowel, Co. Kerry. Natural Foods, 26, Paul St., Cork. Natural Health, Wilton Shopping Centre, Cork. Natural Health, Arthur Quay, Limerick. North Square Pharmacy, Macroom, Co. Cork. Tim O'Malley, Dooradoyle, Limerick. Ormond, M.P.S.I., Cork. Nature's Way, Cork City Car Park. Quigley's Pharmacy, Fermoy, Co. Cork. Jack Shanahan, High St., Killarney. Tralee Health Store, The Mall, Tralee Shopping Centre. Twomey M.P.S.I., Ballyvolane, Cork. Walsh M.P.S.I., Carrigaline, Co. Cork. Walsh M.P.S.I., St. Luke's Pharmacy, Cork. Wood Wolfe, Bridge St., Skibbereen.

Northern Ireland:

Beans'n'Things, 53, Botanic Ave., Belfast. Body Reform, Cornmarket, Belfast.(natural cosmetics) Essentially Pure, 2, Grasmere Gardens, Belfast. (Essential Oils) Food for Thought, 380, Woodstock Rd., Belfast. Health and Herbs, 32, Castle St., Lisburn, Co. Antrim. Iona Shop, 27, Church Road, Holywood, Co. Down. Kiva Oils, P.O.Box 3, Bangor, Co. Down. (Essential oils and unrefined vegetable oils, wholesale). Natural Choice, 217, Kingsway, Dunmurry, Co Fermanagh. Only Natural, 12, Abbey Lane, Armagh. O'Reilly, 9, Townhall St., Enniskillen. Rainbow Health Store, 88, Castle St., Comber, Co. Down. The Wholefood Shop at the Cottown, 88, Cottown Road, Bangor, Co. Down. The Nut-Meg, 9, Lombard St., Belfast, Co. Antrim. Viva Wholefoods, 21, Society St., Coleraine, Co. Derry.

The Irish Association of Health Stores (IAHS)
Current membership is 25 health food stores around the country. Its aims are: to promote better nutrition in Ireland; to promote and protect the interests of Health Store retailers; to maintain and improve the standards of quality, care and service. The IAHS runs training courses and regional seminars.

Committee members are: Roger White, The Nutkeg, Castle Shopping Centre, Swords, Co. Dublin; Tina Kennedy, The Honeypot, Athlone, Co. Westmeath; Derek Kelly, General Health Food Store, Marlborough St., Dublin 1.

Magazines and groups

Earthwatch, The Irish Environmental Magazine
Earthwatch Ltd., Harbour View, Bantry, Co. Cork. Quarterly. Available by subscription, from wholefood shops and some newsagents; articles and facts on environmental and related issues, in Ireland and internationally. Earthwatch campaigns include: Atmosphere, including Greenhouse effect and the Ozone Layer; Acid Rain; Toxics/pesticides.

Watching briefs on: Water Pollution; Nuclear Power; Food Irradiation; Recycling; Tropical Rainforests. There are fifteen local Earthwatch groups, details available from Earthwatch, Bantry. Tel. 027-50968/51283/50545.

The Irish Vegetarian
The Vegetarian Society of Ireland, 31, Pembroke Rd., Ballsbridge, Dublin 4. Quarterly. Recipes, dietary advice and information, animal experimentation and environmental issues, Vegetarian Society news. Activities include cookery demonstrations, Public talks on vegetarianism; Animal Experimentation and related topics; and eating out.

Network
WHANI, 20, Ballybunden Rd., Killinchy, Co. Down BT23 6RD. Quarterly. Annual Subscription: £5stg. or IR£7.50 for four issues. Network is the official organ of WHANI, the Wholistic Health Association of Northern Ireland, a recently formed non-profit making organisation for the promotion of

wholistic activities in the province and throughout Ireland. Articles on Alternative Medicine, Spirituality, Mysticism, Energy, Food, News of Wholistic Health events, activities, centres, etc.

Health and Beauty

Health and Beauty Magazine, 10, Woodford, Brewery Rd., Blackrock, Co. Dublin. Monthly. A glossy, available from bigger newsagents, covering recent developments in natural health therapies and products and giving information on their application and on natural beauty aids.

Health Now

Health Now, Seymour House, South Street, Godalming, Surrey, GU7 1BZ. Quarterly. Advertiser, available free from many chemists and wholefood shops. Covers natural medicines and therapies, recent research, gives recipes using healthy foods, not exclusively macro-biotic.

The Green Guide to Ireland

By John Gormley (Wolfhound Press, 1990). Urgent reading for every man, woman and child. It covers all green issues; air, water and pollution; forestry and bogs; waste and recycling; the household consumer; energy; green holidays; education. A source of reference, information and advice. A practical consumer's handbook and comprehensive citizen's guide to all matters green.